T0220472

The Nation of Nurses

Jalil A. Johnson, PhD, MS, ANP-BC, is an advanced practice nurse, educator, advocate, speaker, and influencer. He is known as a renaissance nurse in that he has broad experience and expertise in many areas, specifically subspecialty areas related to healthcare. He began his career in healthcare in 2000 as a Certified Nursing Assistant and continued his education as an LPN (2001) and RN (2006), completed his nurse practitioner training (2010), and went on to receive his PhD (2018). He is a Hluchyj Fellow (UMass, Amherst, 2012), Facebook Community Leadership Fellow (Palo Alto, California, 2019), and Fellow of Innovation, Entrepreneurship, and Leadership (SONSIEL, 2019).

His clinical practice background includes bedside nursing in ICUs, EDs, telemetry units, and subacute units, as well as long-term care, medical–surgical units, and psychiatric units. His advanced practice experience includes an adult primary care specialty, with subspecialties in behavioral health and substance use disorders. His research experience includes study of the intersection and influence of culture on health disparities in minority populations. His teaching experience includes didactic and clinical teaching at the associate's degree, bachelor's degree, and doctorate of nursing practice level.

His leadership experience includes work as a charge nurse, supervisor, manager, and program director in both inpatient and outpatient settings. He is the CEO of Show Me Your Stethoscope, an online nurse advocacy community of over 600,000 nurses, and an organizer for NursesTakeDC, a grassroots movement of bedside nurses advocating for safe nurse staffing. Professionally, he is most passionate about helping healthcare professionals become greater self-advocates. He is a father to six children, and husband to his wife, who is also a nurse.

The Nation of Nurses

A MANUAL FOR REVOLUTIONIZING HEALTHCARE

Jalil A. Johnson, PhD, MS, ANP-BC

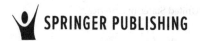 SPRINGER PUBLISHING

Springer Publishing Company, LLC
11 West 42nd Street, New York, NY 10036
www.springerpub.com
connect.springerpub.com/

Acquisitions Editor: Elizabeth Nieginski
Compositor: diacriTech

ISBN: 978-0-8261-5267-1
ebook ISBN: 978-0-8261-5268-8
DOI: 10.1891/9780826152688

21 22 23 24 25 / 5 4 3 2 1

The author and the publisher of this Work have made every effort to use sources believed to be reliable to provide information that is accu-rate and compatible with the standards generally accepted at the time of publication. The author and publisher shall not be liable for any spe-cial, consequential, or exemplary damages resulting, in whole or in part, from the readers' use of, or reliance on, the information contained in this book. The publisher has no responsibility for the persistence or accuracy of URLs for external or third-party Internet websites referred to in this publication and does not guarantee that any content on such websites is, or will remain, accurate or appropriate.

Library of Congress Control Number: 2021907486

Publisher's Note: **New and used products purchased from third-party sellers are not guaranteed for quality, authenticity, or access to any included digital components.**

Printed in the United States of America.

This book is dedicated to all of my ancestors, who sacrificed so much to make my success possible, and to my children, Jenna, Jihan, Alena, Turner, Nora, and Ellis, for whom anything is possible.

Contents

Foreword

Question: How do you plan to engage with the content in this book? There are many ways to digest this information, but as innovators and leaders, a few key paths come to mind. Some of you may read through the eyes of the dreamer. The person who gets inspired by the remarkable lessons within. One who wishes things could be better and envisions what a brighter future might look like.

Others may have the viewpoint of the doer. Someone who interprets this mass of new knowledge as a road map to success. Making lists and checking off the achievements one by one as they're completed (I mean, we are nurses after all).

Both approaches have their own merit, but my challenge for you, the reader, is this: Be the dreamer and the doer, not only in reading this book but in every step you take thereafter. The nursing profession has waited for our permission slip to be innovative leaders for far too long. That mind-set must change, and this book will teach you how. So don't wait for your invitation to lead; get started now (seriously, this very second).

Consider this book your permission slip to make your voice heard. Take risks and try new things. Be the change your patients and communities need. Dream and do. And when you don't get that invite for a seat at the table, as the amazing Shirley Chisholm would urge, BRING A FOLDING CHAIR.

Tim Raderstorf, DNP, RN
Chief Innovation Officer at The Ohio State University College of Nursing
Co-Author of the AJN Book of the Year: *Evidence-Based Leadership, Innovation and Entrepreneurship for Nurses and Healthcare: A Practical Guide to Success*

Preface

The World Health Organization declared 2020 the Year of the Nurse and the Midwife. Indeed, it was the year of the nurse. The entire world's population floundered under the weight of a highly contagious virus. A global pandemic ensued, bringing the world economies to a near standstill. Health systems reached their breaking points and people came to understand, and possibly value, nurses differently. At this crucial time, a nursing shortage looms over our healthcare systems as baby boomers, many of whom are nurses, retire. Nurses are leaving the bedside in droves and the pandemic has pushed many nurses to their breaking points, leading in many cases to early retirement or leaving the profession altogether. I wrote this book as a way to address and combat these problems.

People use the word "potential" when they describe imagined or unimagined possibilities. I wrote this book to describe the potential for nurses, individually and collectively, to completely revolutionize healthcare as we know it. So, in many ways this book is about pathways to accessing the potential of people. This book is equally about the power of community, how communities are

shifting and evolving, and how community is our greatest asset as individual and collective change agents.

The concepts of this possible and preferred future
for nurses and healthcare overall were developed and
inspired by two intersecting parts of my life. My primary
inspiration is from two decades of work in healthcare,
where I practiced and taught nursing at nearly every
level. This somewhat unique experience allowed me various vantage points to view healthcare and nursing. My
experience spans from the student to the professor and
from the certified nursing assistant to the healthcare and
executive leadership table. These experiences heavily
influenced this book and the concepts within.

Additionally, an equally important inspiration for this
book came from the 5 years I spent immersed in a virtual
world with over a half-million healthcare professionals
(primarily nurses) from all around the United States and
many parts of the world. During this time, I was able to
string together what these professionals had in common,
what they struggled with, what they wanted, and where
they fell short. These wonderful and dedicated people
were extremely different from each other in most cases,
yet it was their collective stories that helped develop
the concept of this book and even the title, *The Nation
of Nurses*.

I began thinking about writing this book after I completed my PhD dissertation defense in 2018. Having only
recently completed and published my dissertation, and
with some eagerness to start documenting and collecting ideas about this book, I began writing in 2019 with
the hope of formulating what I thought would be useful
information for any "generic nurse." By 2020, I was well
into writing this book when the COVID-19 pandemic
started sweeping the globe, decimating communities
and healthcare systems alike. As 2020 came to a close, it

became far too clear that nurses everywhere were needed in increasing numbers and that the nursing community would need a better way forward if we were to be prepared for the future.

My primary aim for writing this book is to start a cultural revolution within nursing, and my secondary aim is to create a better, healthier, and more equitable world for all people through the concepts, approaches, tactics, and strategies discussed within these chapters. It is my aim to reach every kind of nurse, practicing in every place, to challenge each of them to make one small, easily outlined, and attainable step toward a better future for us all.

This book is intentionally not an academic venture. I wrote this book in such a way that any and all nurses can access, identify, understand, and implement these concepts and strategies. Additionally, I wrote this book for any type of nursing student, nursing instructor, or professor. Any student nurse, practicing nurse, or even retired nurse can use these concepts to create real positive change within their communities and within healthcare at large. I believe there is something here for every nurse, from novice to expert; we can all benefit from this book.

The global pandemic of 2020 reminded the world of why we value nurses. I appreciate this heightened awareness and spotlight on the value of nurses within the healthcare system. However, science will ultimately prevail, the pandemic will end, and the problems within healthcare and nursing will continue, unless we do something different. I believe this book is that pathway forward. My goal is to put this book in the hands of every practicing nurse and every nursing student and for each one of these people to take one step forward toward a nurse-led healthcare revolution.

Jalil A. Johnson

Abbreviations

AACN	American Association of Colleges of Nursing
AFL-CIO	The American Federation of Labor and Congress of Industrial Organization
ANA	American Nurses Association
CNA	Certified Nursing Assistant
DNP	Doctor of Nursing Practice
FIN	Female IN
GDP	gross domestic product
HCAHPS	Hospital Consumer Assessment of Healthcare Providers and Systems
HMO	health management organizations
IV	intravenous
MNA	Massachusetts Nurses Association
NIH	National Institutes of Health
NP	nurse practitioner
PA	physician assistant
PACU	post anesthesia care units

PPE	personal protective equipment
SMYS	Show Me Your Stethoscope
WHO	World Health Organization

Origins of a Nation of Nurses

INTRODUCTION

I believe that the four million nurses in the United States are carrying the bulk of the healthcare system on their backs; therefore, we (the nurses) should have a significant influence over what happens in healthcare at every level. Full stop. You might be wondering, "Who is this person making such claims and what is this book about?" The short answer is, I am a nurse and this book is about moving the influence of nurses beyond the bedside and giving real pathways that empower the community of nurses to make real systemic change within healthcare. This book is my vision for how we will make this idea a reality. This is important because without a vision we cannot create our preferred future. I believe that as nurses, in our preferred future, we are not only at the decision-making table; we decide how the entire healthcare system functions.

My Start in Healthcare

Throughout my 20-year career, people have asked me a version of the same question: "Did you always want to be a nurse?" Or, worded another way, "Why did you become a nurse?"

I don't think people would ask that question so often had I been a woman; however, as a black man in a profession dominated by women, people ask me this question often. The truth is, I started my healthcare career totally by accident.

I grew up as the oldest of eight children, in a family that survived on an annual income less than $10,000 in the rural south. To say my parents were all consumed with just keeping our family afloat would be an understatement. In that sense, we didn't learn a lot about other aspects of how the world works. Perhaps they thought I was bright enough to piece things together, or maybe they thought that, as their oldest son, I would figure life out. Regardless, I had very little guidance as far as how the real world worked.

After I graduated from high school, I set off into the world without a real plan. I did, however, have a partner. We were young, and not long after we started our relationship, I found myself a 19-year-old father of a baby girl. Throughout my life, my father always had trouble holding down a steady job. I was raised in abject poverty and as a young new father, I promised myself I would never raise a family in that kind of despair.

I worked as many odd jobs as I could. There were so many jobs—working assembly lines in warehouses, maintaining landfills, cutting tobacco, laying sod, serving as a security guard, cleaning bathrooms in office buildings. Honestly, I didn't mind the work as long as I could provide for my family.

The job that changed my life was the one I lost, as in, I was fired. I was working at a restaurant chain as a dishwasher. The work was dirty but honest. I seemed to be treated fair for the most part; the work was 40 hours per week, and it paid nearly $7.00 per hour! This was a total score for a 19-year-old kid in the south!

One fateful evening, I stood in line at the time clock with four other employees, waiting to clock in. The shift manager approached, pointed to each and every one of us and said in a dry, matter-of-fact kind of way, "You, you, you, and you. Y'all can go home."

As the other three started walking away, I asked, "I'll be back tomorrow, OK?"

She responded flatly, "Nah, you don't ever have to come back, I don't need ya."

I stayed and pleaded with her to allow me to stay and work or at least be allowed to come back the next day. I literally begged her, "I'll clean around the dumpsters."

"No."

"Maybe, I'll just hang out just in case you need help later."

"No."

"Please, I really need to work . . . I have a baby at home to take care of."

The manager shrugged her shoulders, lit a cigarette, and blew smoke in my face. She gave me my last warning, "You need to leave, now . . . I don't need ya."

I caught the bus home. I was living check to check, and if I didn't work, there wouldn't be any check coming.

The next day I used some of the last remaining dollars I had to buy a box of ramen noodles, some diapers, and a few cans of tuna. I spent the next few days looking for work but kept coming up short. I was despondent to say the least. On the third day, I kissed my baby goodbye and then told her mother I was leaving and wouldn't be back until I'd figured out how we were going to survive. I gave her 5 of my last 10 dollars and left our apartment, truly unsure of where to go or what to do.

I caught the bus to an area of the city where there were lots of restaurants and strip malls. I filled out applications all day and into the evening. When night came, I was too far from home to walk back and only had $1.75 left in my pocket, and I still had not figured out what I was going to do for a job.

I took a newspaper that was left on a table at a Waffle House I had applied to. I decided to walk through the night for as long as my legs would carry me. When the streetlights would allow enough light, I read the jobs section. There was an ad for free certified nursing assistant (CNA) classes at a local technical school on the other side of town. I walked through the night and slept for a few hours at the back of the school.

I spent the morning and afternoon applying for jobs near the school and at the school. That same evening, I asked the person at the information desk about the CNA program. Great news: The 4-week training was nearly FREE, but there was a catch. I needed to pay for the books. I had no money for books and the next class was starting the next week.

It seemed like a hopeless situation. I left the information booth and sat on a bench in front of the school. The answer to my problems seemed so close, but the roadblocks seemed unrelenting. Even so, I was determined to figure out how to make this work.

As I sat pondering my next move, a man approached me. I must have looked pretty rough—hair in dreadlocks, baggy pants, thin frame, likely a bit dirty and smelly, and a scowl on my face. He asked, "How are you doing? Everything OK?"

I don't know why, but I poured it all out to this man. I told him about my job, my family, that I hadn't really slept last night, that I was hungry. I told him I just wanted to work. He just listened.

Then he pulled out some cash and handed it to me. He said, "Come back tomorrow and ask to speak to Dr. King." I left the school with $17.75 that I'd received from this stranger in my pocket and a lot of uncertainty.

The next morning, I returned to the school and asked for Dr. King. That generous man who had given me his spare change was the dean of the school. He walked me to the financial aid office and asked them to help me complete my financial aid package. He emphasized that I needed to start the upcoming CNA course.

Dr. King didn't mention to anyone how he'd helped me out. In fact, he never mentioned it again. I remember thinking, "If I ever make it, I'm going to help people out the way he helped me."

The next week I met my CNA instructor and began my first experience in healthcare as a CNA student. My instructor had been an LPN for what seemed like 1,000 years. She had worked in the local community hospital ED for over 20 years, until they started phasing out LPNs. Now relegated to less acute clinical settings, which was not her interest, she taught CNA classes as she was nearing retirement.

My instructor approached teaching with gusto! She was energetic, firm, and kind. When I was in high school, teachers and course work were simply throughways to what I really wanted to do—play sports. As an adult learner, my instructor was the first teacher who engaged me in a way that made me feel like I belonged in the room.

After my first day of classes with my instructor, I thought, If I ever get the chance to teach people, I'm going to teach in the same way she taught. I wasn't even sure I wanted to teach, but everything about how she taught seemed right.

After working in hospitals and EDs for most of her career, my instructor really knew her stuff and often reminisced about the good ol' days of "saving lives in the ED." She would go off on tangents as she taught us skills, reminiscing while teaching "hands on" techniques. She seemed to know everything. You couldn't convince me that she wasn't the goddess of nursing.

After a week or so in the classroom and skills lab, my instructor met with me and the three others in my cohort at a large nursing home where we would complete our clinical rotation. We showed up, each dressed in those terrible all white, nearly translucent uniforms, the ones guys wear with the zipper in the front, the flared-out collar, and terrible pleats on the back of the shirt. The uniform was awful and a far cry from anything remotely masculine.

Our instructor gave us our assignments. Some people had more than one person to care for. However, I only had one person to care for during my entire rotation: Darrell.

Darrell, a charming southern man in his 40s, was a practicing Jehovah's Witness. He was neat, organized, and very precise about everything and knew every detail about his care. Darrell was a quadriplegic as a result of a gunshot to the head he had sustained in his early 20s.

Before I met Darrell, my instructor explained many of the things I would need to do to care for him. I'd need to check his blood pressure, set up his food tray, help him get dressed, help him get into his wheelchair, and pretty much do whatever else he needed help with for that day.

My instructor told me Darrell used a Texas catheter and showed me how to apply it, to which I replied, "How am I supposed to put that on a man?"

Honestly, as a heterosexual man who had grown up in a conservative southern culture, I was mortified by the idea of putting a condom on another man. She told me, "Darrel will teach you," and he did. He explained why he was incontinent and how the Texas catheter helped him to be more functional.

Several days a week, for 3 or 4 weeks, I took care of Darrell. I took care of his meals. I checked his vitals. I dressed him in three-piece suits several times a week so he could attend the Kingdom Hall. I learned to use the lift to load him into his chair and did activities with him. I took him out of the chair when he was done with those activities for the day and put him back in bed. I put on his Texas catheter as he instructed me to. He taught me how to do everything to take care of him. I learned how not to tie his shoes too tight because he couldn't feel his feet. I learned how to do some basic range-of-motion exercises to help relieve his muscle spasms. I learned how to bathe him and shave his face. I learned that it was really difficult to dress a 200-pound quadriplegic man in a suit, but it was worth it to him every time. I didn't see much of my instructor during my rotation. She knew Darrell would teach me just about everything I needed to know, and he did.

By the end of my rotation, Darrell and I had grown pretty close. On the last day of my rotation, Darrell told me that over the past 10 years he had not had anyone care for him the way I did. He told me that I was good at this kind of work and to not underestimate how important it was for every person that I would ever care for.

That was that exact moment I realized that whatever difficulty I endured in my duties, they paled in comparison to the impact I could have on the individual, and that caring for other people was what I was meant to do. Most important, I realized that whatever effort I expended in the care of others was truly small compared to the fullness I felt in my heart, knowing I spent my time in the service of others. I realized that the work I was doing really made a difference.

The time I spent with Darrell birthed me into the world of healthcare. I would go on to spend the next 20 years of my career climbing the professional ladder. I became an LPN in 2001 (the most difficult training I've ever completed). I went on to earn an associate degree (RN) in 2006 and a bachelor's degree (BSN) in 2008. I completed my master's degree and training as a nurse practitioner (NP) in 2010. Eventually, I completed my training as a nurse scientist (PhD) in 2018. Along the way I worked in every kind of setting that would have me. I worked as a traveling nurse in ICUs, EDs, postanesthesia care units (PACU), medical–surgical units, substance use treatment areas, home healthcare areas, and behavioral health units. I taught CNAs, LPNs, RNs, and doctor of nursing practice (DNP) students.

I have been caring for people, patients, colleagues, and students with the same intention for the past 20 years and I've never forgotten how amazing it feels to empower someone else. In recent years, I've found myself working as an organizer to support grassroots nursing movements (Show Me Your Stethoscope/Nurses Take DC). I write and speak about empowering nurses as individuals and as a profession at large. My belief is that an empowered nursing profession is the key to revolutionizing healthcare. This idea ultimately became my purpose and life's work. This is my way of giving back to a profession that has given my life so much purpose.

My career in healthcare started without an understanding of my purpose or passion. However, even in my early professional years, I was dedicated to living the old cliché, "Be the change you want to see in the world." My purpose was to be in the service of others. Over time, I would eventually learn that my passion was creating positive cultural and systemic change. That is what this book is about.

A Nation of Nurses

A fair question for you to ask me would be, "What makes me qualified to write this book?" To answer that, I would reply "My background." My opinions and perspectives are the culmination of 20 years of experience as a nurse. I have practiced nursing at several education/training levels and in various settings. Importantly, I have spent the past 4 years being connected to, interacting with, collecting information from, and discussing these topics with hundreds of thousands of nurses from all around the United States and around the world. These experiences had a significant impact on me as a clinician, as an educator, as a nurse scientist, and as a nurse advocate. However, my connection to mass numbers of nurses was as unintentional as my career start.

In 2015, Miss Colorado Kelley Johnson, who also worked as a nurse, gave a monologue during the talent portion of the Miss America beauty pageant. She presented her monologue wearing scrubs and a stethoscope as she described her interactions with a patient and how they were both impacted by the "work." This was surely a proud moment for any nurse viewers. The following day, the panel from a nationally syndicated television show (*The View*) lambasted and insulted Ms. Johnson. They asked, "Why is she wearing a costume?" and "Why is she wearing a doctor's stethoscope?" It wasn't simply the fact that this panel decided to poke fun at an individual. Their insults struck a chord because they indirectly suggested the role of nurses had *less value*, that nurses were no more than *doctor helpers* or *handmaidens*. What they said in no uncertain terms what that the nurse was not even capable of owning a stethoscope. Naturally, nurses around the United States and from around the world were immediately and justifiably outraged. This outrage was palpable throughout the nursing community. Physicians and allied health professionals also joined in. Immediately after the offensive segment on *The View*, social media flooded with nurses expressing their outrage. Sponsors for *The View* pulled their support. Even physicians and allied health professionals expressed their collective outrage. The hashtag #NursesUnite was born and, along with it, the concept of nurses collectively supporting each other.

In response to these volatile comments from *The View* panelist, a bedside nurse from Missouri, Janie Garner, RN, decided to form a virtual community using Facebook groups. Because Missouri was known as the "show me" state and considering the comments from *The View* about Ms. Johnson's stethoscope, Janie Garner called the group Show Me Your Stethoscope.

Within the first day of forming this community, 200,000 members were in the community. That number grew to over 800,000 in its first week. Janie Garner then began assembling her team, trying to figure out what exactly was happening and what to do next.

A nurse friend of mine invited me to the community 3 days after inception. I noticed that there was a lot of positivity and enthusiasm among its members. Nurses shared stories. They discussed the comments from *The View*, but they also just started talking shop. There were stories that ranged from joyous, to terrifying, to all kinds in between.

I also noticed the ugly parts of the nursing culture rear their ugly heads. There were discussions about which nursing subspecialty was most skilled, how much education was needed to be a good nurse, and which shifts did more work.

Without much thought, I·made a post in the community with a photo of myself wearing my stethoscope. My proclamation was simple: I listed my long line of credentials and experiences and acknowledged that I was not better than any other nurse; I believed this community was an opportunity to really do something positive for our profession. Tens of thousands of nurses chimed in and agreed. One of the community moderators suggested I work with Janie Garner to help her organize the community. So, I contacted Janie and we began a relationship that would change our lives and the lives of thousands of people over the course of the next 4 years. The Show Me Your Stethoscope team of bedside nurses went on to connect, engage, empower, and support nurses around the United States and the world. In many ways, this way of mobilizing nurses was unlike anything else nurses had collectively organized. Chapter 6 includes a discussion and some methodology for using virtual communities to engage, empower, and mobilize nurses. This method of using community to mobilize nurses into action was a microcosm of what could be for nursing and for all of healthcare.

Nursing Origins

The nursing profession has been, and continues to be, difficult to define. Contemporary nursing is broad, highly specialized, and complex. It has been called an art and a science, a profession where individuals work to ensure the health and safety of others and the general public

11

through education and compassionate, skilled care. We could easily say nursing as a profession includes some aspects of medicine, social service, and teaching, combined with unique training to engage with individuals throughout the life span.

The nursing scope of practice allows for nurses to care for people throughout their lives, from prenatal care, before we take our first breaths, to hospice care, when we take our last, as well as all arrays of human stages of life in between those ends. Nursing skills range from counseling to improve health literacy to diagnosing and treating complex diseases and includes a plethora of capabilities in between those extremes. Aside from the most influential aspects of the U.S. healthcare system, nurses touch nearly everything in the system.

Modern nursing has evolved to be this way. However, nursing has been practiced in one form or another for thousands of years. There was a time when nursing was only conducted by nuns, other religious women, or the military. Around 1700 CE, nursing was mostly relegated to lower class people. Although someone needed to take care of the sick and infirmed, this was not considered profitable or honorable in the old days. The idea of nurses as healthcare agents capable of making real change in population health outcomes did not arise until the mid-19th century.

By the mid-1800s, Florence Nightingale would begin making her mark and changing the future of healthcare forever. Nightingale was an upper class British social reformer and statistician now known as the founder of modern nursing. During the Crimean War, physicians who treated the wounded would go from soldier to soldier without washing their hands. As a result, most soldiers died of infection rather than their wounds. Nightingale made strides to improve the medical conditions of wounded soldiers by instituting radical practices like handwashing and in the process dramatically reduced the mortality rates for wounded soldiers.

You may be wondering, "Why are we talking about a British socialite from the 1800s?" Nightingale didn't just "do a job" or care for people, like most nurses; rather, she fixed problems. She was innovative, creative, and bold. In 1870, she wrote, "It will take 150 years for the world to see the kind of nursing I envision." Nightingale would go on to give us many pearls. Similar to today's modern nurses, the nursing profession faced staffing shortages in the 1800s. To that point, Nightingale wrote, "To increase the efficiency of this class [nurses], and to make as many of them as possible the disciples of the true doctrine of health, would be a great national work" (Nightingale, 1860, p. 79).

The contemporary nurse must combat pseudoscientific ideas undermining the health of populations (i.e., anti-vaccination movement). Nightingale encouraged us to use evidence to guide practice, proclaiming, "The most important practical lesson that can be given to nurses is to teach them what to observe—how to observe—what symptoms indicate improvement—what the reverse—which are of importance—which are of none—which are the evidence of neglect—and of what kind of neglect" (Nightingale, 1860, p. 59).

The modern nurse is often spread so thin in their practice. Often, the balance of life and death rests between a great catch and a small mistake, a missed observation or a hurried save. Nightingale reminds us that the safety of our patients depends on us being available and present, "If you look into reports of trials or accidents, and especially of suicides . . . it is almost incredible how often the whole thing turns upon something which has happened because 'he,' or still oftener 'she,' was not there" (Nightingale, 1860, p. 22). Surely, Nightingale was ahead of her time as we still grapple with some of the problems she discussed 150 years ago.

The World Health Organization proclaimed 2020 as the Year of the Nurse. Coincidentally, that year marked 150 years from Nightingale's prediction. I will not prophesize Nightingale's words; however, while nursing began as a task-oriented job for poor people to care for other sick or infirmed people, the profession has evolved substantially from its origins. The contemporary "idea" of a nurse still holds mythical and angelic properties. Surely, there are laypeople who envision nurses as women with little white hats employed to hold patients' hands and get coffee for physicians. However, in reality, over the past centuries we've seen modern nursing evolve and develop from "hands on" training taught by physicians to diploma programs, and ultimately to the professional degrees, many specialty certificate programs, and even more specialties and subspecialties. We are, in fact, independent thinkers, innovators, and lifesavers.

Still, in the year 2020, nurses continued to strike at community hospitals. Global pandemics like COVID-19 ravage healthcare systems. This pandemic killed hundreds of nurses, while healthcare facilities struggled to provide basic personal protective equipment (PPE) to their nursing staff.

I often wrestle with, and now ask you to also ponder, this simple question: "Why are nurses struggling with the same problems Nightingale wrote about 150 years ago?" Specifically, how is it that 150 years have passed and we are still debating how to effectively staff a facility, or trying to figure out how to produce enough competent nurses to care for the population, or how to take care of patients without hurting the staff? Did Nightingale's vision come to fruition? These are the questions we must ask ourselves as individuals and as a profession.

Finding Purpose

In my early years as an APRN, I worked at an outpatient clinic providing care to underserved populations. In this clinic, 80% of the patients identified as Hispanic. Of those patients, 90% identified as Puerto Rican. I noticed that some health outcomes specifically related to noncommunicable diseases were not very good in this clinic. Other healthcare providers (nurses, physicians, etc.) also noticed this.

Specifically, I could not understand why, despite our best efforts, we didn't do a great job of helping people control type 2 diabetes. In this particular state where I worked, everyone had access to health insurance. Many of the patients spoke English and interpreters were always available for those who spoke English as a second language.

I thought if these are the standard medical treatments for this condition, why aren't our patients getting better? As I was preparing my doctoral work and learning to be a scientist, I thought this was a problem worth investigating. Over the course of several years I conducted a deep dive into the subject, asking the question, "Why aren't we doing a good job helping these particular patients?"

I conducted a qualitative study to examine the cultural variables affecting self-care for Puerto Rican–identified individuals with type 2 diabetes. I interviewed nurses and physicians as well as patients at our clinic and individuals in the community. I spent 3 years reading everything I could on and around the subject of type 2 diabetes management and Hispanic populations. I spent over 2 years conducting the study. At the conclusion of the study, I found there were powerful cultural variables and influences affecting self-care that we, as healthcare providers, did not account for, were not aware of, and almost never discussed with our patients. I found that as a healthcare community, we were not providing culturally competent and culturally relevant care to our patients, and our outcomes were proof of our oversight (the results of this study are published and publicly available at the University of Massachusetts, Amherst). Importantly, our treatments and interventions could not and would not be effective because we did not understand or consider the culture of the people we were trying to help.

Conducting this study affected the way I view problems. I learned that if a tactic and strategy are typically effective but ineffective in a certain population, we should examine the tactics and strategy as well as understand the culture of the population we're trying to help. We must understand before we can provide solutions.

In some ways similar to the patient population I was trying to understand in my study, the nursing profession is not doing well. We could even say the nursing profession has a chronic kind of illness: a complex, poorly understood, all-encompassing kind of illness.

Perhaps you may wonder, "How can a profession be sick?" For argument's sake, let's define a chronic illness as a persistent or otherwise long-lasting condition/disease that affects health. This "professional disease" has deep social, cultural, and economic roots. For example, the nursing profession has the greatest number of people supporting the healthcare system but has the least effective voice when it comes to making systemic change. Nurse-to-patient ratios are so high we are not able to provide quality care in the way in which we were trained. Subsequently, nurses must literally "hack" around systems to provide care. We have a culture of lateral violence that is deep and entrenched within our ranks. In addition, violence toward nurses and healthcare providers is on the rise, with no real solution in place. There is a culture of retaliation from our employers toward nurses who speak out. New graduate nurses are graduating and literally thrown to the wolves to care for patients who are sicker than they've ever been. Nurses are not viewed as authorities on healthcare and have almost no presence in media as such.

An illness typically has symptoms. For example, consider that one out of every three new graduate nurses will leave the bedside within the first 2 years due to burnout. A nursing shortage looms as the baby boomers retire. Burnout and compassion fatigue are common. The depression rate for nurses is double the national average across all professions (9% general population, 18% nurses). In some ways, the nursing profession is literally causing the illness and the symptoms.

This way of defining the nursing profession as having a chronic illness with symptoms may seem overwhelming. As an individual nurse, a student nurse, or a person in the public, you may ask, "What can I do about those huge problems?" Perhaps after reading this list of problems, you may even think, "How can I help if I don't fully understand those problems?"

As with many chronic illnesses, optimal health can be achieved and restored. However, we must first understand the problems. The next step is to treat the problems with real and practical solutions. Finally, we must use tactics and strategies to maintain optimal health.

Tactics and strategies have been used to improve the nursing profession and move nurses from apprentice-like handmaidens, to highly skilled autonomous practitioners who save lives. However, the tactics used to empower nurses to fix the problems in the nursing profession and the healthcare system at large have essentially been a Band-Aid on a gushing wound.

In this book I discuss the problems listed earlier. I also discuss less understood problems such as how reimbursement systems affect the nursing profession as well as cultural factors that undermine the nursing profession.

Additionally, the following chapters are discussions on many of the issues within the nursing profession and within healthcare as they are experienced by nurses. We will take a deeper dive into the culture that causes these problems. Finally, throughout this book, I offer real and practical solutions every nurse can use to address these problems.

- Chapter 2 is a discussion of nursing and politics. Here I discuss the effect of mainstream political discord on nurse self-advocacy as well as how nurses are changing this.
- Chapter 3 includes a discussion of systemic problems within nursing education as well as solutions.
- Chapter 4 is a discussion of the flaws of the U.S. healthcare model, specifically the model of reimbursement as it relates to nurses and the nursing profession.
- Chapter 5 is a discussion of nurse leadership and empowerment opportunities.
- Chapter 6 is a discussion of mobilizing nurses to be self-advocates in various modalities and trends and opportunities in new markets as well as practical and innovative solutions.
- Chapter 7 is a discussion and a summary of recommendations for driving nursing influence, the revolutionary potential of nurses, and a vision of the future of nursing and healthcare at large.

I wrote this book for a broad audience, including student nurses, practicing nurses, nurse educators, and the public. I believe that in order to change our future we must empower future nurses. We must also provide real and practical solutions for practicing nurses. Finally, we must pull the public into these conversations, as the public will ultimately bear the brunt of the problems we discuss.

Throughout my 20-year career I have completed six nursing programs. As a student, I learned basic principles of how to take care of people and communities. I learned how to manage people, patients, and conditions. Each time I received new training, I reentered the workforce with renewed purpose. However, I learned nothing about the culture within the nursing profession. Importantly, I was not told that nurses were a community of change agents, nor was I informed of any specific pathways to engage in the community of nurses.

Over the course of my career I was never informed that nurses COULD and SHOULD change everything about healthcare to make it work better. In my training years, I was told very little about how the healthcare system works. I was taught almost nothing about the problems within the healthcare system. I was never told that this scope of change was our responsibility. I would learn much of this information through trial and error, through hundreds of interactions and connections, slowly and often painfully over the course of my career. I wrote this book for every nursing student and every practicing nurse, irrespective of level of education, specialty, or practice type. If I had read this book earlier in my career it would have completely changed my career and everything I understood about nursing.

This book is also written for the public. The public perception of nursing does not reflect the training and experience needed for nurses and the ever-so-essential nursing workforce. Nurses are commonly depicted in media as task-oriented "physician helpers." The plight of the nurse is largely unseen by the public. However, nurses' concerns have direct implications on how the public receives care. Considering that nearly every person at some point between life and death will require nursing care, it is imperative that the public understand that they should be very concerned about the nurses' concerns.

Lastly, this book is for anyone who cares about transforming healthcare, grassroots organizing, and establishing equity in the workplace. The U.S. healthcare system is a large, complicated, multibillion-dollar industry. The chase for profits has obscured the quality of the care healthcare providers can give and the quality of the environments in which they practice. The advent of social media and the rapidly expanding age of information allow for practitioners to truly leverage their numbers and expertise to make change. Nursing, a profession dominated by women, is largely undervalued, which is evident from the consistent reports from nurses. Throughout this book I discuss these issues along with real practical solutions, as well as a vision for how nurses can use these tactics to revolutionize the healthcare system.

PRINCIPLES AND METHODOLOGY

Nurses are well positioned to reclaim the healthcare industry and put the care back in healthcare. Nurses are painfully aware of the issues within the nursing profession as well as broader systemic issues. However, beyond the bedside most nurses are not active as change agents when it comes to broader health policy. Importantly, nurse participation in self-advocacy varies greatly.

This book is built on three principles: storytelling, the ladder of engagement, and the snowflake model.

Storytelling

Storytelling is a powerful tool, showing that influence and knowhow are transferable and every nurse can have influence beyond the bedside. Storytelling is one of the oldest and most familiar ways we communicate as humans. Stories allow each of us to give context, pass on valuable information, and influence people. Stories are often interwoven within our lives. Grandparents tell us stories of the old days. When we court our partners, we tell stories of our past and present and eventually talk about the future story we'd like to be a part of. We tell our children stories to illustrate a point, drive home a lesson, and sometimes just to make them laugh. We tell stories when spending time with friends to help them get caught up on our lives.

Stories can also be very powerful tools when crafting a story of the nurse. We can use stories when trying to influence each other and the public. Throughout this book, we will reexamine storytelling as a method to influence and empower. Storytelling is a complex art form. I suggest this simple format—story of self, story of us, and story of now. This is a reliable and concise method for using stories as a way to mobilize and influence.

Story of Self

The "story of self" is an introduction to who you are. It humanizes the writer and allows the reader to connect on a personal level. For example, if I write to an audience of nurses, I might write, "My name is Jalil. I have been a nurse for 20 years."

Story of Us

The "story of us" unites the writer and the reader. This is an opportunity to connect with the reader. If I continue the previous story, I might write, "Unsafe staffing puts patients at risk and leads to burnout. Unsafe staffing is a huge problem for nurses and the reason I left bedside nursing. In the midst of a nursing shortage, many nurses are leaving the bedside for the same reason, but I think we can unite to fix this problem."

Story of Now

The "story of now" is a call for action. It is based on the story of us, takes the points made, and creates an actionable plan. To finish the previous story, I might write, "I believe nurses can help make policy to address unsafe staffing. I wrote this petition asking my congressional representative to draft legislation addressing unsafe hospital staffing. Let's make this happen together. Please sign and share this petition with your friends and family."

As a narrative, the story reads,

> My name is Jalil. I have been practicing as a nurse for 20 years. Unsafe staffing puts patients at risk and leads to burnout. Unsafe staffing is a huge problem for nurses and the reason I left bedside nursing. In the midst of a nursing shortage many nurses are leaving the bedside for the same reason, but I think we can unite to fix this problem. I believe nurses can help make policy to address unsafe staffing. I wrote this petition asking my congressional representative to draft legislation addressing unsafe hospital staffing. Let's make this happen together. Please sign and share this petition with your friends and family.

Ladder of Engagement

The ladder of engagement is based on the idea that every nurse can have influence beyond the bedside. The "ladder" is figurative and represents levels of engagement. It is a way to conceptualize how the entire population of nurses can be mobilized and engage in self-advocacy. With the advent of the ever-evolving reach of social media platforms, nurses generally fall into one of six categories in terms of advocacy for nursing and healthcare issues.

These categories, or levels, are as follows: activist, highly engaged, moderately engaged, minimally engaged, aware, unengaged, and the unaware. The categories can be defined as shown in Table 1.1.

Most nurses fall into one or two of these categories. So, we can figuratively place all four million nurses in one or two of these categories. To visualize this, we can place the 1% to 3% of nurses participating in leadership or self-advocacy as activist at the top of the ladder. The other

Table 1.1 Levels of Engagement	
Level 6: Activist	Change agents directly engaged in advocacy, policy making, and creating dialogue; these individuals are highly visible entrepreneurs, innovators, and leaders who create engagement opportunities for self and others and seek out and engage issues
Level 5: Highly engaged	Seek out opportunities to engage online; likely to engage in person; will participate if the pathway is created; seek out and addresses issues
Level 4: Moderately engaged	Passively engaged online; may participate in an in-person event if convenient
Level 3: Minimally engaged	Unlikely to engage online; may participate in online activities if convenient
Level 2: Aware, unengaged	Aware of the issues; do not participate in addressing them
Level 1: Unaware	Unaware of the issues or have accepted the status (students, novices)

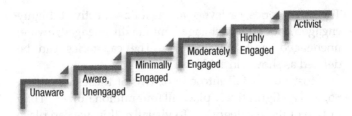

Figure 1.1 Levels of engagement ladder.

categories follow, stepwise, concluding with the unaware nurses (students, etc.) at the bottom (Figure 1.1).

To mobilize the entire population of nurses as self-advocates, we must meet each nurse where they are on the ladder of engagement, provide them with a suitable way of engaging, and help them move to the next rung. For example, a student may not be aware of the problem or complexity of the problems associated with violence against nurses in the workplace. By educating all student nurses about the subject, we've met them in a suitable environment and moved them up from the first level (unaware).

Snowflake Model

The snowflake model (not to be confused with the slur for easily offended people) is based off of the idea that influence and knowhow can be transferred from one person to the next. This snowflake helps illustrate the concept.

The center is a tight network of connections. Each connection leads to more connections and so on and so forth. In this model, a person at the center has influence and knowhow. This person can influence and empower each of the people they're connected to in the next outer ring, and each of those people can influence and empower each of the people they're connected to, and so on and so forth. Connecting several snowflakes together forms a network.

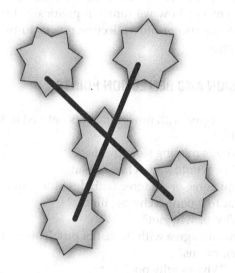

CONCLUSION

Chapter 1 covers a lot of ground. We discussed some pertinent origins of the nursing profession, defined nursing practice and evolution of practice, explained the origins of some key concepts, lightly touched on some of the common problems, and introduced the key principles and methodology.

Nursing has evolved as a profession, yet we (nurses) have been struggling with some of the same problems for over 150 years. In the history of nursing, we have not capitalized on our collective political, cultural, and social power. As we move through the chapters, please consider these points, principles, and methodologies.

In the next chapter, we jump right into nurses in media and politics. Politics can be a sore topic. However, in order to make change in nursing we must first understand the culture of dysfunction. We must understand who we are and how we function politically. Only then can we make use of our collective power to make systemic change.

DISCUSSION AND REFLECTION POINTS

1. Do you agree with how nursing is defined in this chapter?
   a. What's missing from this list?
   b. How would you define nursing?
2. Do you agree or disagree with describing nursing as similar to having a chronic illness?
   a. Why, or why not?
   b. Do you agree with the list of problems and symptoms?
      — Why or why not?
   c. Are there other problems you would include?
      — Why or why not?
3. Try to write a short but compelling story (any story) using the framework detailed in the chapter.
   a. Story of self
   b. Story of us
   c. Story of now

4. Tell a story about nursing using the story of self, us, and now.
5. Where do you fall on the ladder of engagement?
   a. When it comes to healthcare?
   b. When it comes to issues in the nursing profession?
6. Reflect on the snowflake model. Try to remember an instance when it was used.
   a. Did anyone inspire or empower you in your career?
   b. If so, did you then go on to inspire and empower others?
   c. If so, did those people go on to inspire others?

REFERENCE

Nightingale, F. (1860). *Notes on nursing*. D. Appleton and Company.

2

Underrepresentation and Politics

INTRODUCTION

Take a moment and imagine the last time you saw a nurse on television, in a movie, or in the news. Did you view the nurse in a movie, on television, or on social media? If the nurse was in the news, was it local, national, or international news? What was the role of the nurse? Were they a main character? Were they a hero, a side character, or a villain? If you are a nurse or nursing student, did you see yourself reflected in this character? If so, was it accurate? Keep these questions in mind throughout this chapter.

If you've taken so much as a fifth-grade history class in the U.S. public school system, you have learned about the Boston Tea Party. You can probably remember images in textbooks of men, dressed as Native Americans, tossing boxes of tea into the Boston Harbor. Their gripe was that they were being taxed by the English kingdom, and they had no say in the matter. The notion of taxation without representation was unfair and we, as a nation, would not stand for it. This, among other provocations, would eventually lead to the Revolutionary War, a conflict uniting the colonies and eventual leading to foundation of the United States. A founding principle of Western democracy is being led by a representative government. If you live in the continental United States, you are probably under the assumption that the elected government officials represent you and your interests. Take a moment and think of an influential government official. Is this person a nurse or healthcare provider? If not, think of any government official who is a nurse or healthcare provider. If no individual comes to mind, ponder that throughout the discussion in this chapter.

In this chapter, we examine representation of the nurse in media and politics. As you read through the chapter, reflect on your experiences and political affiliations. Try to picture how you, your employer, and your community fit into the scenarios.

MEDIA AND ONSCREEN

I will admit, I've binge-watched many episodes of *House*, and nearly all of *Grey's Anatomy*, with my wife, who is also a nurse. We absolutely love these shows. *House* is a medical drama based in a hospital setting. The main character, Dr. House, is a drug-addicted genius physician who leads a team of other genius physicians as they solve medical mysteries. *Grey's Anatomy* is one of the longest running and most popular medical-based dramas. The main character, Dr. Meredith Grey, is a talented surgeon. Much of the show surrounds her personal life and work at a level 1 trauma center.

Anyone who has ever been to a hospital, especially a trauma center, knows the buildings are literally full of nurses. However, the nurses of *Grey's Anatomy* and *House* are only seen in the background, occasionally responding, "Yes, right away doctor," as physicians scream orders and do nearly all of the work of saving lives. I cringe every time I watch a physician on these shows ambulate a patient, administer and teach them how to take their oral medications, transport them around the hospital, and start peripheral intravenous (IVs). Physicians *can* do all of those things; however, and quite frankly, they don't. In nearly all hospitals, nurses do those jobs, and many other jobs being carried out by the physicians in *Grey's Anatomy* and *House*.

The many stereotypes of nurses on screen, if they are seen, are often portrayed as the trusty and obedient doctor's helper, or even the villain. It is easy to understand why the public is fascinated with physicians on screen. Physicians are a rare people, with a knowledge base to which most people are drawn. I would argue that nurses are equally as interesting and four times as common, and yet, nurses are rarely depicted as central characters.

Despite nurses being relatively absent on screen and in the media, the public still trusts nurses, specifically when it comes to honesty and ethical standards. Nursing has been voted the most trusted profession for the past 18 years running. A multitude of nurses have had a family member or friend share some personal details in hopes of getting some free, confidential, and reliable medical advice.

We should ask ourselves, "Why is a profession dominated by women not worth exploring? Are nurses not championed on screen because the profession is so serious? Is the entire profession, broad and encompassing as it is, completely void of heroes? Is nursing boring?" The truth is there's no shortage of content or stories; every nurse knows the job is anything but boring. I cannot count how many times I've heard a nurse colleague say, "We should make a show about this; no one would believe this happens in real life."

The downstream effects of pop culture are powerful, and these stereotypes are harmful beyond nurses getting visibility or positive roles on screen. They undermine the intelligence and aptitude of the nurse and paint the nurse as a second-class profession. The media encourages the next generation to dream big and become change agents in the world, while simultaneously dissuading them from joining the ranks of nurses as a real meaningful way to change the world. It is no surprise that when young people are inspired to change the world, they don't consider becoming a nurse as a means to do so.

These stereotypes relegate nurses to background figures. They undermine the true impact that nurses can have at and away from the bedside, and dismiss the idea that the largest workforce in healthcare can and should drive the system. Ultimately, this leads to a public that may trust nurses, but doesn't naturally turn to nurses to fix the problems in healthcare.

Nurses in the News

Can you remember the last time a nurse was in the local, national, or international news? Typically, nurses make the local news after some atrocity. You're more likely to see a headline that says "Nurse Abuses Patients at Nursing Home" than you are to see "Nurse Creates Life-Saving Device." Nurses are nonexistent in the national news.

The Woodhull study on nursing and the media, originally published in 1998, examined how frequently nurses were used as primary sources in news and news related to health. They found that less than 1% of articles in major news sources referenced a nurse; and nurses were referenced in less than 4% of health-related articles (GW Nursing, n.d.). This study was replicated by Mason et al. (2018), and the findings showed not much has changed. Prior to the COVID-19 pandemic of 2020, only 2% of news articles include nurses as sources and nurses were never the source in stories on health policy.

Naturally, we do not want negative stories of nurses becoming the norm. However, what about the news covering health? Healthcare is a hot topic for local, national, and international news regarding health crises and healthcare policy. There is no good reason why there are not more nurse and nursing perspectives represented in the news.

We have 24-hour news coverage of every kind of news. From international catastrophic events to local tragedies, there is no end to the stream of news coming our way. Social media allows the public access to all of the news, and it is accessible all the time. Not a day passes without a report of a violent conflict affecting thousands, or a weather event that displaces a community, or new and emerging public disease concerns. Yet nurses are on the ground and involved in all these cases. Nurses will receive and care for the patients after a bombing. After a mass casualty incident on a local highway, it will be nurses who receive these people in their local hospitals and care for them. When Ebola rears its ugly head in the Congo, it will be the local nurses on the front lines caring for people. The "nurses" are not just present in these stories; they are an essential component in the stories. The fact that the perspectives and contributions of nurses to these stories are omitted is problematic beyond getting due recognition for "doing the work." It means the nurses are literally unseen, and, thus, their perspectives and contributions are unnecessary.

The downstream effects of the culture of excluding nurses from media are that the public does not seek out the nursing perspective. In the public view, nurses are an afterthought when it comes to solving systemic healthcare problems. As far as the public is concerned, the nurses are not the hero in any story beyond the bedside.

Actionable Steps: Underrepresentation in Media

The nurses' collective preferred future should be that nurses are trusted and valued beyond the bedside. How we are perceived by the media has a direct effect on how the public perceives nurses. It would be impractical to direct producers of movies and television to elevate the role of the nurse on screen and in the news. However, art imitates life. In order to be included in media, we have to change the way producers of art see "real life." We must reinsert ourselves into media by creating cultural change, thereby changing the public perception of "a nurse." We must standardize and write our own narrative of who the nurse is, what the nurse knows, what the nurse does, and what the nurse can do.

Challenging the Narrative

My wife, Kate, is considered a "millennial." Like others of her generation, she prefers online shopping to visiting department stores. She is no recluse; she just prefers to read reviews from other consumers before committing to a product. This trend of purchasing based on consumer feedback is powerful and only getting stronger as more and more tech savvy consumers enter the market.

Writing an honest review is not only helpful for fellow consumers; it has immense power for the base of consumers. Most people will overlook a single negative review. They are savvy enough to see past a single data point. However, a cluster of negative reviews is highly suggestive to a consumer. Online entertainment platforms like IMDb and Rotten Tomatoes as well as public social media profiles allow nurses to speak directly and give valuable feedback to the public and other consumers.

In order to change public perception, we must standardize the narrative that nurses will challenge and critique their presence or absence in media and that misrepresentation or underrepresentation are distorted truth. As a profession, we need to get used to asking questions like, "Where is the nurse in this story? Are the nurses represented accurately? Does this undermine the value of my profession?"

We should share the answers to these questions publicly with the aim of provoking conversation. These are some ways every nurse can influence the public and media markets as well as challenge and change the narrative of the nurse as a background or less useful character on screen and in media.

As a general approach, all nursing students, practicing nurses, and retired nurses should be critical and vocal about low visibility and mischaracterization of nurses in film and media. There are many ways for nurses to influence media and film. Storytelling is a way for nurses to use their influence. Methods may include letters, email, and social media platforms. Please refer to the levels of engagement ladder for the rest of this section (see Figure 1.1).

Practicing nurses should use both active and passive approaches to increasing positive visibility of nurses in the news. Passive approaches may include being vocal about issues within their communities and sharing their perspectives "as a nurse." Active approaches may include learning media communication skills, offering themselves as topical experts, and, to a lesser degree, sharing concerns directly to media outlets.

Engaging the Problem

Depending on the level of engagement, there are ways for every nurse to challenge misrepresentation and under-representation of nurses in media and on screen.

Level 1: Unaware

People at level 1 of engagement should be made aware of the low visibility and misrepresentation of nurses on screen. These include nursing students and novice nurses. Every nursing curriculum should include discussions on the low visibility of nurses on screen as well as specific methods of offering public critique. Graduates should be encouraged to be critical and vocal about how nurses are portrayed in film and in the media.

Preceptorship is an excellent time to impart knowledge as well as the realities of nursing on a new nurse. Experienced nurses should discuss the lack of accurate nurse representation with novice nurses. Additionally, they should encourage new nurses to be vocal and express their opinions publicly.

Level 2: Aware, Unengaged

People at level 2 of engagement are typically practicing nurses. They are aware of the low visibility and misrepresentation of nurses on screen. However, they rarely participate in addressing this problem. Nurses at this level of engagement should use social media platforms and online rating systems to offer online critiques of media and news outlets.

Level 3: Minimally Engaged

People at level 3 tend to be savvy with their online critiques but tend to engage only when convenient. These nurses should seek out opportunities to offer online critiques of media and TV outlets where nurses are misrepresented or underrepresented.

Level 4: Moderately Engaged

People engaged at level 4 passively engage online and may participate in nurse advocacy in person if convenient. These nurses should offer online critiques and seek out opportunities to be more vocal. Additionally, they should encourage nurses in their networks to be vocal about misrepresentation and underrepresentation of nurses in media and on screen.

Level 5: Highly Engaged

People engaged at level 5 seek out issues online, are likely to engage in person, and tend to participate if there are no barriers. These nurses should offer online critiques, seek out opportunities to be more vocal, and encourage others to be more vocal about misrepresentation and underrepresentation of nurses in media and on screen. Additionally, these nurses should add storytelling to create dialogue with colleagues and the public. Finally, these nurses should write articles and offer heavy critiques regarding underrepresentation or misrepresentation of nurses in media and on screen.

Level 6: Activist

People engaging at level 6 are change agents and social influencers. These nurses tend to be highly visible entrepreneurs, innovators, and leaders, and include those in political office, high level executives, prominent academics, and social media influencers.

These nurses should offer online critiques, seek out opportunities to be more vocal, and encourage others to be more vocal. They should also use storytelling to create dialogue with colleagues and the public, write articles, and offer heavy critiques. Finally, these nurses should use, create, and empower networks of nurses to address this problem; and use their influence to stimulate calls to action in the form of online critiques and petitions.

Professional Organizations

As representatives of the nursing disciplines' profession, nursing organizations have an opportunity to champion nurses beyond the bedside. All professional nursing organizations should support and champion positive representations of nurses in media, on film, and in the news. Affirmation of authenticity goes a long way in the hearts and minds of artists. Additionally, professional nursing organizations hold news outlets accountable for excluding the nurse perspective and are especially critical when news outlets exclude nurses when reporting on health-related information, news, and policy. Nursing organizations are responsible for driving the push for fair nurse representation in media and on screen. Nurses should be highly critical of professional nursing organizations that do not champion nurses in media and on screen.

Academic Institutions

Nursing schools are extremely influential as faculty have an opportunity to shape nursing beyond the bedside. Nursing faculty should push for their curriculum to include discussion about the lack of nurse representation in media as well as include basic communication and media training. Furthermore, basic higher education for nurses should teach and encourage nurses to report on issues and to be the voice of healthcare beyond the bedside. Nurse educators should offer health-media training for practicing nurses interested in being correspondents and experts for media outlets.

POLITICS

Nurses feel unseen because we are literally unseen in the political arena. One major complaint nurses report is feeling as if the work, and perspective, of the nurse is undervalued. There are sociocultural reasons for this, including longstanding patriarchal attitudes about a profession dominated by women. Let's discuss how this plays out at a systemic level.

Many of the professional and occupational problems nurses struggle with are related to healthcare policy. Few nurses are active at the policymaking level, and even fewer are influential. Nurses feel underappreciated and undervalued because the people designing healthcare are not nurses and do not consider nurses or the nurse perspective on healthcare. Healthcare design is directly influenced by healthcare policy, which is made by politicians, and there are almost no nurses in political office.

Politics can be very difficult to discuss. The nursing profession is socioculturally, demographically, and politically diverse. Therefore, nurses don't have a sociopolitical "view" when it comes to policy. However, nurses should have a way of approaching politics and policy. There is a pathway to this "nurse view" of politics and policy; but first, let us talk about the issues that divide us.

Political Discord

Take a moment and remember the last time you had a disagreement with someone about a political topic. Were you among friends or family members? Was it at work or in a professional space? Was it in person or online? Was it casual, lighthearted, or funny? Did you or the other person get angry? Did you feel better after the conversation? Remember this moment, and the specifics of the situation. We will circle back to this experience later.

There may not be a single topic more divisive than modern politics. As professionals, we've been trained to avoid discussing politics in the workplace. Over the past decade, the age of information, 24-hour news, and social media has pushed politics front and center in our lives. We cannot escape the news, the events, the information about every detailed win or loss from our elected officials.

The major political points our elected leaders squabble over have entered our lives in such a way that we cannot help but form opinions on the topics. Yet it is often considered taboo to discuss politics at work or at family gatherings. Perhaps common decency and the likelihood of disagreement suggest we avoid the political topics and just "get along."

Common decency and manners notwithstanding, political discord has always been heavy in the United States, with major and minor parties constantly vying for power and control of the three branches of our government. Throughout the 1850s, U.S. political power would settle into one of two major parties (Democrats and Republicans). While there were and still are many minor parties (Libertarian Party, Green Party, etc.), these two parties generally still hold the most political power in the U.S. political system.

The contemporary versions of the two-party system in the United States are fairly dogmatic and divided on their approach to policy. Generally, the parties will use a conservative or a progressive approach, with the current version of the Republican Party leaning conservative and the Democratic Party leaning progressive.

Conservative approaches generally lean toward less regulation and progressive ideas generally lean toward government regulation and oversight. Candidates seeking election will discuss these major issues as talking points throughout every national and state campaign.

The Pew Research Center (Bialik, 2019) lists the top public issues, in order of importance, as the (a) economy, (b) healthcare costs, (c) education, (d) terrorism, (e) Social Security, (f) Medicare, (g) poor and needy,

(h) immigration, (i) jobs, (j) reducing crime, (k) drug addiction, (l) budget deficit, (m) race relations, (n) military, (o) transpiration, (p) climate change, and (q) global trade. For argument's sake, let's agree that nurses should be concerned with the economy, healthcare costs, education, Social Security, Medicare, the poor and needy, reducing crime, drug addiction, and race relations.

Education

Nurses should be concerned with education policy. A population with low literacy will have even lower health literacy. The work of nurses often involves educating a person on how to stay alive, despite a health condition that may otherwise kill them. In these cases, a patient's life depends on their literacy.

Medicare/Medicaid

Hospitals and clinics are filled with the chronically infirmed, older adults, and people with disabilities. Many of these patients are surviving on Social Security benefits and receive Medicare health coverage. Importantly, the idea of a government-funded public healthcare option (Medicare for all) is a hot topic with ongoing political and private debate. If implemented, this idea will have massive systemic impacts. Nurses should be concerned with policy affecting Medicare and Medicaid.

Social Problems and Addiction

Many communities, from affluent suburbs to inner city slums, have populations who have been affected by addiction. While the most recent opiate epidemic has crept into wealthier communities, many poor communities have been struggling with the problems surrounding addiction for decades. Nurses should be invested in these issues as the people affected will eventually be our patients.

Race Relations

Health disparities have existed in the United States for hundreds of years. Native American tribes, enslaved Africans, and most recently Hispanic immigrants, among many others, have experienced negative health outcomes directly correlated with government policies. There have always been segments of the U.S. population experiencing poor health outcomes compared to the general population. Nurses, being acutely aware of health disparities, should be concerned with policy that further marginalizes or improves outcomes for affected communities.

The most divisive political topics include the economy, abortion, gun laws, immigration, healthcare, and climate change. Considering nearly all U.S. citizens will eventually become patients, nurses should be concerned about the economy. Nurses, as frontline clinicians managing these problems, are acutely aware of policy surrounding reproductive health, including abortion and access to contraception. As such, nurses should be interested and vocal about their positions.

The nursing profession is diverse and prevalent throughout many parts of the United States. Some communities are greatly affected by gun violence while others are not. Regardless, nurses should formulate and share opinions on any policy affecting gun ownership and access. Nurses care for vulnerable populations, including immigrants. Nurses should be concerned about policy affecting immigration. Finally, nurses should obviously be concerned with healthcare politics and policy.

Economy

The United States has the largest and most robust economy in the world with a gross domestic product (GDP) of $19.39 trillion (2019). The modern U.S. economy is robust enough to sustain an over two-decade war in the Middle East (1990 to present) and the housing crisis and recession of 2008, which nearly crippled the world economy. Over the past decades, U.S. wages have not risen with inflation, the culture of lifelong employees is dead, and nearly an entire generation has crippling student loan debt. On a positive note, immediately prior to the global recession caused by the COVID-19 pandemic of 2020, unemployment in the United States hit a record low of 3.5% in 2019. Still, the economy and availability of good jobs is a top priority for U.S. families. Those who support conservative economic policy tend to support free market economic models and reduction of tax burden to boost business/growth, while those who support progressive economic policy tend to support government investment in infrastructure and education, entitlement programs for those in need, and industry regulation.

Most nurses are considered "middle class" and are affected by the ebb and flow of the economy. Naturally, we should be concerned about economic policy. The economy also has an effect on our patients. The hierarchy of needs tells us that when resources are low, people will prioritize preserving and sustaining life over general health and well-being.

Abortion

The landmark *Roe v. Wade* Supreme Court decision pushed the abortion debate front and center in U.S. politics. Those who support conservative policy tend to lean toward pro-life policy and do not support abortion. People supporting progressive policy tend to support pro-choice policy, and with it, the right to choose an abortion. There are many reasons why a person may choose to support or oppose policy on abortion.

Second Amendment

The Second Amendment of the U.S. Constitution allows citizens the right to bear arms. The debate over interpretation of this amendment is especially contentious, considering the longstanding culture of firearm ownership in parts of the country, prevalence of firearms, deaths by firearms, and routine mass shootings. People who support conservative policy tend to support the right to bear arms, whereas people who support progressive policy tend to support government regulation of firearms.

Immigration

The United States, although considered a "nation of immigrants," has a long history of political discord surrounding immigration. From the original Europeans who landed on the eastern shores and the ensuing problems with Native Americans; to the millions of enslaved Africans who endured 400 years of oppression; to the waves of Europeans, seeking a better life; to the most recent immigrants from the southern border—each wave of people faced condemnation and scrutiny. People who support conservative policy tend to support stronger border security and control (e.g., former president Donald Trump's border wall), while people who support progressive policy tend to support immigration reform, including an easier pathway to citizenship.

Healthcare

There are numerous issues within the healthcare industry, including but not limited to rising costs (pharmaceuticals, insurance, administrative, etc.); poor access to quality care; health disparities; and labor shortages. People who support conservative policy tend to lean toward approaches that reduce industry regulation and rely on the free market economy, while people who support progressive policy tend to support expansion of entitlement programs (Medicare, Medicaid), industry oversight/regulation, government options (i.e., Affordable Care Act, a.k.a. Obamacare), and collective bargaining organizations.

Climate Change

The climate change debate is relatively new to U.S. politics. There is scientific consensus (97%) that climate change is real and that the phenomenon is affecting weather patterns. The debate has fallen to deciding whether or not there are ways to combat the phenomena; what, if any, government policy should be enacted to combat the phenomena; and if the phenomena was caused by human activity. More and more of the public is concluding that climate change is real. However, how much of the global warming and weather events are related to human activity and what, if anything, can be done to stop these phenomena remain up for debate. The current debate appears to fall along partisan lines, with conservatives questioning drastic regulation targeting industry and progressives more in favor of sweeping overhaul of industries thought to be contributing to climate change.

These are some of the common political issues, but this list is not exhaustive. The point here isn't to give every nurse a political science degree, nor is it to tell a nurse how to vote and what political stance to align with. Quite frankly, there are many other issues people care about. Regardless of how we came to develop our political stances on the issues, these issues are the ones that stir us up and awaken our passions. These are the issues that we tend to choose sides about, and the ones we rarely ever change our positions on.

At the beginning of this section, I asked you to recall the last time you discussed politics with someone who disagreed with your point of view. Perhaps, politically, you lean conservative and were speaking to someone who leans progressive, or vice versa. Recall this moment again and try to answer these questions:

- Was the topic one of those listed earlier, or something else?
- Were you among friends or family members?
- Was the conversation at work or in a professional space?
- Was the conversation in person or online?
- Was the conversation casual, lighthearted, or funny?
- Was the conversation tense or emotional?
- Did you or the other person strongly disagree with each other?
- Did you or the other person get angry?
- Did you feel better after the conversation?
- Did either of you change your stance on the topic?
- Did either of your "facts" change the conversation?
- Who won the debate?

If you had the experience most people have in these situations, of course the person did not change their stance from progressive to conservative, or vice versa, and neither of you "won" the debate. There are many reasons for this. We can call it cognitive dissonance, confirmation bias, motivated reasoning, and so on. Simply put, it is human nature to convince ourselves that opposing ideas, and the people who hold them, are ignorant, crazy, immoral, bad, stupid, or all of these. The single most reliable point that both parties can probably agree on in these debates is the fact that people do not like to change their minds or beliefs. In politics, beliefs in ideas are all that matters. I would venture to say the key to winning as a politician is not to convince people to believe what you believe; the key is to convince them that their beliefs align with yours. Divisiveness is a strategy that helps politicians win elections. A politician must separate themselves from opposing candidates and convince a large enough segment of the population to vote them into office.

Why does the way politicians operate to win votes matter? Politics may be complicated, but the answer to this question is simple—politics drives policy, and policy affects people. Nurses are in the business of helping people; some would argue nurses have a passion for it. Policy, especially healthcare-related policy, directly affects the work we do, how we do our work, and all the lives we touch throughout our careers. More importantly, if nurses are to truly revolutionize the nursing profession and healthcare, political influence is one of the surest ways to transform policy.

Politically, aside from being dominated by women, nurses are not a homogeneous group. In fact, the U.S. nursing profession has a great deal of sociocultural diversity, which may include individuals' political, geographic, racial, ethnic, and socioeconomic backgrounds. Politically, there may be some predictability on how a population may vote. However, nurses typically vote along the lines of their sociocultural and socioeconomic communities.

Pick any of the controversial political topics listed earlier. There isn't a single one where nurses vote or choose candidates reliably in the same way, not one where nurses have influence, not one where the "nurse vote" is considered essential. When a politician seeks election, nurses are not considered an essential population worth targeting; as such, they are not viewed as needed to make policy change. The people who make general policy do not care about the nurse's opinion. These are the same people who make healthcare policy. The net result is that healthcare policy does not consider the nurse view; subsequently, nurses feel unseen, unheard, and undervalued. The problem of nurses not being considered as a voting block translates directly to nursing and healthcare policy as well as the corporatization and dehumanization of the healthcare industry.

Political Identity

When I started working with and talking to hundreds of thousands of nurses online, there was an overwhelming call for nurses to mobilize and "do something" to change healthcare for the better. Although there was some agreement about how to make those changes, what was most evident was how divided people were politically. For years I pondered this problem—how do we make nurses a voting block?

This question made me ponder how I saw nurses politically, and how I saw myself politically. I would like to think that I define myself in terms of plurality. For example, I could say that I am male, of African descent (primarily), a father, a husband, a brother, a scientist, a nurse, a leader, a teacher, an activist, a writer, and so on. I could go on and on. The point is, when we really think about what defines us, it is not based in singularity. We are more than the culmination of our gender, sexual orientation, relationship status, income, job, career, race, ethnicity, citizenship, activities, family, and so on. Yet at times we define ourselves with singularity, with a primary identity and secondary identities to follow.

What part of our identity gets us off our feet and motivates us to stand up and do something? Often it is the primary identity that drives what we care about. This does not mean that we don't care about anything outside of our primary identity, but our primary identity can be a driver for what we put our energy toward. For example, let's consider three nurses I know personally who work on a medical surgical unit. The first person primarily identifies as a mother and cares about community safety, autonomy to choose schools, and anything that may have a direct impact on her family. The second person identifies as a transgender man, and is very concerned about safety as well, but in a different context as the concerns are related to discrimination and physical violence related to their gender. This person is concerned about safety, but more concerned with policies that affect their rights. The third person is an avid hunter. He is concerned with safety, autonomy, and rights, but perhaps under a different context as they pertain to the Second Amendment and the right to bear arms.

These three nurses have political affiliations that span the gamut from ultra-progressive to far right conservative. They have three different primary identities and may differ greatly as far as what they care about in relation to those identities. They may spend nearly as much of their awake time with their workmates as they would with their families.

The transgender man votes on a progressive ticket to support progressive policies they find beneficial and inclusive of the LGBTQ community. The hunter votes on a conservative ticket to support politicians who oppose the regulation of firearms. The mother may be independent and vote both ways depending on how it affects her family.

Yet these three nurses have the same job and work in the same place. They know each other and their work well.

They all agree that their hospital staffing creates unsafe conditions for patients and staff; and agree that external pressure is required to improve the conditions. However, because political discussion is considered taboo at work, they do not discuss the candidates, nor how or why they have chosen to vote for their preferred candidate. They do not discuss the candidates' position on the hospital staffing problem they agree on. When it is time to vote, they vote along party lines. A politician is elected, and the three nurses go on complaining about the unsafe staffing problem that was not addressed. Regardless of which political party wins, the nurses go on spending most of their days feeling disempowered, unseen, and unappreciated. This divisive way of thinking about politics is how the power of four million nurses gets diluted.

There are many reasons for nurses to be divided. However, there are also ways to unify, empower, and broaden the influence of the profession. Tactics for expanding nurse influence beyond the bedside include storytelling (both intra-professionally and extra-professionally); deconstructing barriers to nurse unity; increasing involvement in political campaigns; forming coalitions; grassroots organizing; and self-advocacy.

ACTIONABLE STEPS: UNDERREPRESENTATION IN POLITICS

Stick With the Science

Contrary to popular belief, as nurses, we do not blindly follow the orders of physicians. We think critically about our work. We use science and evidence to justify our actions, or inactions. I would go so far as to say you cannot be a nurse without believing in the power of science. It is literally our job to be a consumer of, and/or a creator of, science. Our training teaches us to believe in and use science at the bedside. If we want to unify politically, we have to change our professional culture. In order to have impact beyond the bedsides, we have to change the culture around what it means to be a nurse and how we intersect with the consumption and production of science. In our professional roles, we understand how a beta-blocker affects the body, and our practice reflects this; when our patients are using these medications, we check the heart rate and evaluate for hypotension.

We do not form opinions about the pharmacokinetics and pharmacodynamics of medications; we use the most current evidence to decide how to properly care for our patients. Many nurses should be avid consumers and believers in science. This is a culture that we must make sure continues to be instilled within the profession, at the bedside and beyond. After all, understanding and consuming medical knowledge and evidence is our bread and butter. As a profession, we should use this same scientific approach to politics and policy. We should use the most current conclusions of scientific exploration and rigorous studies to determine our actions.

Take, for example, abortion, a typically divisive issue with people choosing their political candidates depending on their position on abortion. For many single-issue voters, a political candidate's stance on abortion is the deciding factor in whether that candidate gets their vote or not. For the sake of argument, let's hold any religious convictions until the end of this section. Let's also set aside any conspiracy theories, preconceived sociocultural bias, and any partisan rhetoric, and simply ask the question—what does the science say?

According to the Centers for Disease Control and Prevention, the number of abortions is in steady decline, 11.6 abortions per 1,000 women age 15 to 44 (Jatlaoui et al., 2019). The majority of abortions in 2016 (the time of the study) took place early in gestation: 91.0% of abortions were performed at ≤13 weeks' gestation; and many fewer (1.2%) were performed at ≥21 weeks' gestation (Jatlaoui et al., 2019).

Fifty-nine percent of women had one or more live births; 41% had no previous live births; 43% of women had one previous abortion; and 56% of women had no previous abortion (Jatlaoui et al., 2019). A reason for the decline in abortions is likely related to multiple factors, including the growing use of long-term contraceptive methods (Nash & Dreweke, 2019). Women in their 20s account for the majority of abortions, and have the highest abortion rates (those aged 20–24 and 25–29 accounted for 30% and 28% of all reported abortions, respectively) (Jatlaoui et al., 2019). According to the Pew Research Center, one in five children is living in a single parent home (Livingston, 2018a), and 30% of single mothers and their families live in poverty (Livingston, 2018a). There is much more data available. However, we can draw some conclusions from this information. The data tell a story. The abortion rate is in decline. Ninety percent of abortions happen before 13 weeks' gestation (late term abortions are rare and usually of medical necessity to save the life of the mother or if the fetus is not viable). Abortion rates are similar for women who have previously conceived and women who have not conceived prior. Women in their 20s account for most abortions. One in five parents in the United States are single, and 30% of them live below the poverty line.

When I summarize this data, I'm reminded of something my 90-year-old grandmother, who is a religious woman, once said: "Every generation has tried to stop the next from having sex, and not one has ever succeeded." My grandmother believes abortion is wrong, albeit legal.

This is what the evidence tells us about the realities of the abortion debate.

1. In a democratic society, we cannot impose our beliefs about morality and sex on others.
2. We, as a society, cannot realistically stop young people from having sex.
3. People are aware that life may be difficult if they have children before they are prepared.
4. Single parents are at high risk for poverty and all the subsequent sequelae.
5. Contraception prevents abortion.

Most nurses agree that our job is to care for the people and the public, regardless of whether we agree with their decisions. As nurses, we should consider the principles of harm reduction, do no harm, and choose the least invasive intervention to treat a problem. Our goal should be to reduce the need for abortions, unwanted pregnancies, and unintended single-parent households. Given the facts and science, an obvious solution is to ensure that people have more than adequate education and access to contraception. This solution would satisfy most people who have pro-life or pro-choice beliefs as it would minimize the need for and number of abortions.

Now, let's translate this directly to politics and policy. Hypothetically, let's imagine local candidates running for state office. The nurses in this district unify on this point and vow to individually and collectively support the candidate who proposes the best policy that offers expanded education and access to contraception. The nurses' campaign, independently and collectively, to support their candidate.

This idea and approach are not an automatic home run. However, it does take the 18-year-long trust the public has given to nurses (as the most trusted profession) and allows them to mobilize and capitalize on this trust and improve the healthcare system as well as public health.

As with most controversial topics, even if there is scientific consensus, there will be outliers who disagree with the evidence. Moreover, there will be conspiracy theorists and people with entrenched ideas. And yes, some of these people will be nurses. Still, it is our job as nurses, and as a profession, to use our critical thinking and training to evaluate the evidence before proposing a solution to a problem.

For example, there is scientific consensus that the climate is changing because of human actions or inactions. Yet the decisions as to whether to support or get behind initiatives to fight climate change are large and divided along party lines. When nurses stop supporting science, we stop thinking like nurses; we resort to political rhetoric and throw all our critical thinking skills out of the door.

The same scientific method used to determine that a beta-blocker slows and strengthens the heartbeat is the same rigorous method used to determine that humans are affecting the Earth's climate, and that this warming is bad for the planet and bad for humans. Nurses should be invested in the climate change discussion because this is a public health issue. Some would argue that it is the greatest public health issue our species will ever face.

Similarly, with other conspiracy theories and hoaxes like the anti-vaccination movement, there should be no question as to where nurses' opinions are regarding vaccinations. There will be some outliers, conspiracy theorists, and people who do not believe in science. That is just human nature. However, the public should know that nurses unequivocally support the current evidence about vaccines—which is that they are more beneficial than they are harmful.

I have seen educated seasoned nurses go toe to toe with other nurses about whether vaccines are harmful. Or whether vaccines cause autism. In the age of information, we have witnessed misinformation spread to hundreds of thousands, even millions, of people. As nurses, we must have a unified stance when it comes to science and evidence.

Nursing is a science that allows for intuition and experience, but our practice and how we think through problems is based on evidence and scientific consensus. Using science is our bread and butter. Beyond the bedside, there will be times when the scientific consensus challenges what we believe or have been taught to believe. In these situations, we tend to gravitate toward like-minded people who agree with our view. After all, it is much easier than being wrong. As individual nurses and as a profession, we must change this culture from within. When our ideas are challenged, we must think like scientists. If a scientist's idea is challenged or disproved, they have two options: (a) Accept that the new idea is more valid than their own, or (b) use better science to disprove the new idea. Simply put, if we do not like the scientific consensus, we should either make a more scientifically sound argument or reconsider our ideas. Nurses should use this same way of thinking beyond the bedside when faced with political or policy questions by asking the questions (a) "Do I accept the scientific consensus?" (b) "If not, why don't I accept the scientific consensus? Is there better science available that disproves the scientific consensus?"

To think like a nurse is to think like a scientist. We can and should use science beyond the bedside to help navigate politics and policy. If we do this collectively, we will become powerful voting blocs. The first order of business when creating voting blocs is to show up as a nurse.

Show Up as a Nurse

If nurses want to have influence in politics and/or influence policy, the first order of business is to "show up as a nurse." Extending nurses' influence beyond the bedside means being a visible constituent. Nurses do not need permission to speak on behalf of nurses or the nursing profession. Nurses aren't in the public eye beyond the bedside. This is one of the great barriers to expanding their influence.

There is a phenomenon in business, academia, and public office where nurses working beyond the bedside supposedly stop identifying as nurses in the sense that they do not lead with "nurse" as their primary professional identity. They may identify as a professor, an entrepreneur, or a public official, but rarely as a nurse primarily. There are many reasons for this. A colleague, who has over 20 years' experience as an entrepreneur and inventor in the healthcare space, once told me he didn't include RN in his credentials or pitches because people wouldn't take him seriously if they knew he was a nurse. This one person alone connected with countless investors, corporations, organizations, and people in his community. Yet most of the people he connected with did not associate his brilliance, perspectives, or achievements with the nursing profession. Effectively, his decision not to disclose his nursing background limited the view of his colleagues. It is plausible that their knowledge of his background could have challenged their assumptions about the contributions of nurses in their spaces, and even inspired them to seek more connections with nurses.

If we compare this phenomenon of nurses distancing themselves from the profession as they move away from the bedside with our physician colleagues, the inverse is true. When physicians move into work away from the bedside, they tend to pull their professional status forward. Beyond that, in their social circles their opinions as physicians are respected, even if the opinion is not in their area of expertise. This is not a critique of physicians, but rather a critique of nursing culture.

When nurses are engaged with the public beyond the bedside it is essential that they identify as nurses. Nurses are the largest workforce in healthcare. By pulling their professional nurse status into their personal and public networks and interactions, nurses effectively change the narrative of who nurses are, what they believe, and how they think. Most importantly, changing this culture within the profession expands the trust and influence of the nurse beyond the bedside.

Voting Blocs

A voting bloc is a group of people who are motivated by a specific common concern; these concerns tend to inform their voting patterns and leads them to vote similarly to each other in elections. Voting blocs may be based on sociocultural, socioeconomic, religious, ethnic, and racial reasons. They can also be related topically. For example, white evangelicals may oppose abortion and tend to vote on the conservative ticket. Political campaigns attempt to convince large swaths of constituents that they not only understand their concerns but that their candidate is the right person to address them. Therefore, it is common, especially in national elections, for candidates to field questions about what they will do to help veterans or minority groups, how they will create jobs, and so on.

There are millions of nurses (~3 million RNs and ~ 700,000 LPNs) working throughout and propping up the U.S. healthcare system. Nurses can use the power of collective numbers combined with longstanding public trust to become a powerful voting bloc. Previously, we discussed how to find consensus on difficult political topics. The next step is to mobilize at the grassroots and national levels.

Micro Voting Blocs

Grassroots organizing can be a heavy lift, but it doesn't have to be. Personal relationships and local communities offer an opportunity to spread influence without getting into large-scale organizing. This is a way to form micro voting blocs. For example, nurses live in several communities: work colleagues, family, friends and social groups, and general community.

In the workplace, nurses can start by discussing political topics with colleagues, find common ground as nurses, and empower each other to form local nurse constituencies around political topics. Each nurse who joins a constituency should bring other nurses into the fold, and so on and so forth.

Within families, nurses can use their influence by sharing the nurse view on a political topic. Nurses should then show up, with their nurses' constituencies, and engage in local campaigns as nurses (e.g., town hall meetings). Nurses should engage with their local organizations to help champion the nurse view of a political problem.

Macro Voting Blocs

Engaged and influential nurses can help drive discussion to find common ground. Using the snowflake model of empowerment, nurses can form local nurse constituencies, which allow for state and regional constituencies. Influential and highly engaged nurses should combine their influence and empower local constituencies to encourage discussion with communities as well as recruit other nurses into the constituency. Nurse influencers should encourage local constituencies to form regional and national constituencies and engage in regional and national campaigns. Highly engaged nurses should run for political office (as a nurse) and lead regional and national campaigns based on the nurse view of a political problem.

Engaging the Problem

Here are some specific ways nurses at each level of engagement can do their part to increase the influence of nurses beyond the bedside. Please refer to Table 2.1 through the rest of this section.

Table 2.1 Engaging Nurses in Media and Politics

Media	Politics	Level 1	Level 2	Level 3	Level 4	Level 5	Level 6 x
Understand issues	Understand issues	+	+	+	+	+	+
Online critique	Work discuss		+	+	+	+	+
Seek engagement opportunities	Online In person			+	+	+	+
Storytelling and create dialogue	Micro bloc Storytelling				+	+	+
Formal articles	Macro bloc Storytelling					+	+
Calls to action	Call to action Politician						+

Level 1: Unaware—Understand the Issues

People at level 1 of engagement should be made aware of the lack of nurse influence in politics and development of policy. Every nursing curriculum should include discussion on key local and national political topics. Graduates should be encouraged to discuss policy as nurses in their work environments and communities as well as in local and national political discussions.

Level 2: Aware, Unengaged—Discuss Issues in Community

People at level 2 of engagement are typically aware of the political problems being discussed locally and nationally. However, they rarely participate in addressing these problems as nurses. These nurses should engage in discussions about policy with their work mates, friends, and family.

Level 3: Minimally Engaged—Activate Online and in Person

People at level 3 are aware of the lack of nurse influence on policy and tend to share their political ideas if prompted. Nurses at this level are unlikely to share their views as a nurse. At this level of engagement, nurses should seek out opportunities to engage and discuss politics and policy with other nurses in their community and online. Additionally, nurses at this level should seek out opportunities to engage in discussion about politics and policy as a nurse with their families and people in their communities.

Level 4: Moderately Engaged—Form Micro Blocs, Storytelling, Engage Policy Makers

People engaged at level 4 are likely to discuss politics and policy online and in person if prompted. People at this level of engagement should initiate political discussion as a nurse with their colleagues, family, and friends and within their community. Additionally, these nurses should initiate micro blocs or coalitions of nurses within their places of employment and communities. These micro blocs should engage, as nurses, with local and regional policy makers. Finally, these nurses empower other nurses by sharing their insight, progress, methods, and challenges online through storytelling.

Level 5: Highly Engaged—Form Macro Blocs, Storytelling, Engage Policy Makers

People engaged at level 5 seek out political discussion as nurses, online and in person. They are likely to push through barriers to self-advocacy. These nurses should seek out and help organize nurse coalitions or micro blocs into macro blocs as well as facilitate the consensus of the macro blocs to policy makers (e.g., attend town halls). Additionally, these nurses should empower other nurses by sharing their insight, progress, methods, and challenges online through storytelling.

Level 6: Activist—Create Pathways to Affect Change; Empower, Promote, and Encourage Voting Blocs; Become Politicians

People engaged at level 6 are highly visible entrepreneurs, innovators, and leaders. They are change agents directly engaged in advocacy, policy making, and creating dialogue and include those in political office, high level executives, prominent academics, and social media influencers.

These nurses should use their influences to create dialogue and pathways to affect change. They should lend their influence on regional and national nurse coalitions (macro blocs) as well as consider seeking political office as nurses.

Professional Organizations

In the 2016 presidential election, the two largest and most powerful professional nursing organizations endorsed presidential candidates. The American Nurses Association offered official support for Hillary Clinton and National Nurses United offered their support for Bernie Sanders, effectively dividing the nursing profession at the highest level. Neither Sanders nor Clinton won the presidency. However, the act of endorsing presidential candidates, especially in a contentious national election, infuriated many nurses.

Professional nursing organizations should not decide the nurse view of policy, nor should they endorse candidates. Instead, they should reflect the consensus of local and national nurse coalitions as well as the science on the issue. Professional organizations empower individual nurses, the nursing profession, and the public by reporting the views and perspectives of local and national nurse coalitions.

Academic Institutions

Nursing schools have an opportunity to shape individual nurses and the profession beyond the bedside. Nursing curricula should include discussion about pertinent local and national political issues as well as the current science on the topics. Importantly, nurse training should include how to think beyond the bedside about politics and policy as well as the implications for not engaging with policy makers.

CONCLUSION

In this chapter, we covered the underrepresentation of nurses in media and politics, the consequences of these problems, and steps nurses can take to come together and correct this imbalance. Additionally, we discussed a nurse-centric approach to political topics and policy. These fundamental principles allow each nurse to view social problems and healthcare through a similar lens and ultimately provide a pathway for nurses to unify and effectively make positive change in healthcare, local and national public policy, and the world. Chapter 3 presents a discussion about nursing education as an institution, and what we can do to make it better.

DISCUSSION AND REFLECTION POINTS
Media and Onscreen

1. What are some examples of underrepresentation of nurses in media and the news?
2. Are there any other reasons why nurses are under-represented in media and onscreen?
3. What is your level of engagement to increase representation of nurses in media and onscreen?
   a. What actionable steps can you take to increase representation of nurses in media and onscreen?

Politics

1. Are you affiliated with a political party? If so, which party?
2. Which of the key issues are most important to you and why?
   a. What does science tell us about this problem and what is the nurse view of this problem?
3. Did the discussion about divisiveness help you in the way you discuss political and policy issues?
   a. Why did this help?
   b. Why didn't this help?
4. What is your "primary identity"?
   a. Does this identity inform your view of politics, politicians, and policy?
5. What is your level of engagement regarding increasing nurse influence on politics and policy?
   a. What actionable steps can you take to increase nurse influence on politics and policy?

REFERENCES

Bialik, K. (2019). *State of the Union 2019: How Americans see major national issues.* https://www.pewresearch.org/fact-tank/2019/02/04/state-of-the-union-2019-how-americans-see-major-national-issues

GW Nursing. (n. d.). *The Woodhull Study revisited: Nurses' representation in health news media.* https://nursing.gwu.edu/woodhull-study-revisited

Jatlaoui, T. C., Eckhaus, L., Mandel, M. G., Nguyen, A., Oduyebo, T., Petersen, E., & Whiteman, M. K. (2019). Abortion surveillance—United States, 2016. *Surveillance Summaries, 68*(11), 1–41. http://dx.doi.org/10.15585/mmwr.ss6811a1

Livingston, G. (2018a). *About one-third of U.S. children are living with an unmarried parent.* https://www.pewresearch.org/fact-tank/2018/04/27/about-one-third-of-u-s-children-are-living-with-an-unmarried-parent

Livingston, G. (2018b). *The changing profile of unmarried parents: A growing share are living with a partner.* https://www.pewsocialtrends.org/2018/04/25/the-changing-profile-of-unmarried-parents

Mason, D. J., Nixon, L., Glickstein, B., Han, S., Westphaln, K., & Carter, L. (2018). The Woodhull Study revisited: Nurses' representation in health news media 20 years later. *Journal of Nursing Scholarship, 50*(6), 694–704. http://dx.doi.org/10.1111/jnu.12429

Nash, E., & Dreweke, J. (2019). The U.S. abortion rate continues to drop: Once again, state abortion restrictions are not the main driver. *Guttmacher Policy Review, 22,* 41–48. https://www.guttmacher.org/gpr/2019/09/us-abortion-rate-continues-drop-once-again-state-abortion-restrictions-are-not-main

3

Nursing Education: Systemic Issues

INTRODUCTION

Nursing is a unique profession in that there are multiple entry points and levels of education associated with nursing. This has certainly allowed the profession to be accessible to people throughout the world, from all walks of life, and of many socioeconomic and sociocultural backgrounds. Unfortunately, within this relatively accessible profession are cultural practices and norms that undermine nursing students, novice nurses, seasoned nurses, and the profession at large. In this chapter we discuss the problems with some of these deeply embedded and negative cultural practices within nursing education as well as solutions to move the entire body of nurses and educators toward a more unified and functional profession.

MY EXPERIENCE AS A STUDENT

In my first semester as an LPN student I received a low grade on an anatomy exam. When I met with my instructor, she pointedly suggested, "Nursing isn't a good fit for you. You should consider one of the trades, like auto-diesel mechanic." For a microsecond, I was disheartened; then, I was angry. I could not understand how a teacher could be so mean. I could not understand why this teacher was giving up on me so easily, or why she assumed so much about me, or why she didn't offer to help me learn. I replied to her question, "No thank you. I think I need to study more." She replied, "Fine, you'll learn the hard way. Suit yourself." To say this teacher was less than supportive of my efforts over the term would be an understatement. Fifty percent of my class did not make it through the program; I did. Some years later after I completed my associate degree and became an RN, I visited my former LPN school, my teachers, and the dean of students. The dean asked if I'd say a few words at the upcoming graduation ceremony, and I agreed.

My talk was brief. I found my teachers, including the mean one, in the crowd. I talked about overcoming adversity, and how hard work beats talent. As I ended my remarks, I looked directly at my former mean teacher and said, "As people who have achieved success, we should be cautious never to gloat or look disparagingly on others. It is our duty to empower and lift others seeking to improve their condition by offering a helping hand." People cheered and clapped, but my mean teacher did not. Momentarily, I felt as if I'd won, as if I had proven something to her. However, after I exited the stage and shook a few hands, I realized I had in fact not won. The mean teacher was still working at the school. Her years of tormenting students were far from over. This was the first time I thought about how bizarre nursing education can be. I would go on to encounter other teachers like this, and each time I thought, this kind of behavior shouldn't be allowed in any profession centered on caring and compassion.

I completed my nurse practitioner (NP) training at a school with three graduate programs: the School of Medicine, the Graduate School of Nursing, and the School of Biomedical Sciences. Medical students and NP students shared some of the same labs and experiences. Part of our NP training involved a transitional course, clearing us to move from classroom learning to community practicum with real patients. One of our tasks was to complete a simulated patient care experience called the OSCE (Objective Simulated Clinical Examination). This "experience" included a video-recorded clinical encounter with an actor in a simulated "doctor's office" environment. It was described as a one-shot deal with no do overs. If we did not pass the exam, we failed the course and could not move on to clinical training. We were terrified of failing the exam. One of my classmates asked a particularly tough instructor, "What happens if I perform the steps of an abdominal exam out of order?" The instructor replied, "Oh, you better not perform an abdominal exam out of order, because if you do . . . ." She didn't say exactly what would happen, but the insinuation was that we would fail the exam and the course. We were told to show up, dress professional, and essentially perform a perfect patient encounter.

On the day of the exam, we marched over in groups and waited our turn. While we were waiting to take our exam, a medical student (studying to become a physician) showed up and jumped the line of waiting NP students. She was wearing flip flops, cut-off jean shorts, and a spaghetti string top. She explained that she forgot to take the simulation exam, and that Dr. so and so sent her over to get it done. My first thought was, surely, she won't pass the exam. She wasn't even dressed properly. I was angered by my next thought—she was clearly having a different educational experience than we were.

A couple of the students had panic attacks. One student got a minor head laceration when she nervously whacked her head into a cabinet during the exam. Nonetheless, she completed the exam, holding pressure on the injury while she did so. We all passed. Still, I was angry. At our debriefing, our instructor asked, "How do you all feel?" Nearly everyone said they were relieved. I raised my hand and replied, "I feel terrible. I can't believe I paid this school money to make me feel terrible for no reason at all." Awkward silence followed.

This was the first time I realized that the mean girl culture I experienced in LPN school was pervasive throughout nursing education. I did not take issue with the difficulty of the exam; rather, my issue was that there was no benefit to the way the teacher made us feel. I imagined her teachers berated her and made her feel small. I imagine the behavior was also passed on to the students, some of whom would go on to be the same kind of teacher. Mostly, I imagined a better, healthier culture in which nurses could learn how to be nurses as well as how to teach nurses.

Nursing education only offers a brief glimpse into advocacy, and it is predominantly focused on advocating for the patient. Generally, we are not taught to advocate for ourselves, for our profession, or to improve the healthcare system. Throughout my career I completed several nursing programs. At the completion of these programs I felt generally prepared to practice and to take my licensing exams. However, I learned very little about how the healthcare system actually works, problems within the healthcare system, or universal problems nurses experience within the system. Furthermore, I wasn't introduced to the concepts of nursing as a community or nurses as change agents beyond the bedside, and I certainly wasn't informed that I had any responsibility or ability to change the healthcare system. Nursing schools have an opportunity to shape a powerful force of empowered change agents. Unfortunately, there are several intra-discipline cultural barriers that prevent this from happening.

Hierarchical Learning

The U.S. healthcare system is hierarchical. Similarly, nursing is a hierarchical profession. Nurses have moved the profession from occupational or skilled labor to a profession with unique depth and breadth of practice. A certified nurse assistant certificate (weeks of training), a bachelor's degree in nursing (4-year degree), and a doctor of nursing practice (DNP) degree (graduate level advanced practice) all allow a person to practice a level of nursing.

Health outcomes and safety improve when nurses advance their education (DiMattio & Spegman, 2019). The American Association of Colleges of Nursing (AACN, 2019) encourages employers to foster practice environments that embrace lifelong learning and offer incentives for RNs seeking to advance their education to the baccalaureate and higher degree levels. There is also an unspoken idea that more education makes a better nurse. Culturally, this could be misconstrued as "value," as if a nurse with more education is more valuable or provides more value. This culture is problematic.

A nurse scientist with a PhD does not necessarily provide more value than a nursing assistant providing hygiene care to an incontinent patient on a night-shift in a nursing home. The roles and functions may be different, but the value does not change with education. The millions of patients in long-term care facilities would agree that their caretakers add much value to their lives. It is safe to say most of these patients would find zero value in a nursing professor. Likewise, nurse scientists are extremely valuable to nursing programs that have a research focus. These programs would find little value in an experienced certified nurse assistant. This is because value is relative to the situation. The value we ascribe to a nurse is also tied to revenue generation. An RN with a bachelor's degree working as a flight nurse is linked to a high price tag care modality, with reimbursement for services reaching into the millions for a single patient. Compare that treatment modality to an LPN working in a long-term care facility, where reimbursement for care barely covers the cost of the services provided, and one could assume the flight nurse is more valuable. In the course of a day the skill of a flight nurse may save several lives, and without care from the nightshift nurse, dozens may die. The value ascribed to reimbursement does not equate to the value of care given or received.

The consequence of a professional culture that equates education and revenue generation with value is that it undermines the true value of every nurse. It reinforces paternalistic ideas that some jobs in healthcare are more valuable than others. It is the embodiment of the phrase "just a nurse."

From the inception of the nursing profession, nurses have been chasing, refining, and honing the idea of the professional nurse. We created training programs, hospital-based diplomas, practical nursing programs, associate degrees, bachelor's degrees, and master's degrees as well as practice and research doctoral pro-grams. Indeed, we have achieved a variety of practice levels for the professional nurse. We also, albeit inad-vertently, created a culture that says loudly and boldly "more education makes a better nurse." Moreover, this culture essentially relegates the responsibility of creating systemic change to the most educated within our profession. Nursing programs typically don't discuss leadership unless the student is in a bachelor's-level program or higher. Nursing programs typically don't discuss system management and theories of change unless the student is in a master's level program. Nursing programs typically don't discuss using evidence beyond the bedside unless the student is in a master's or doctoral level program.

An argument can be made that nursing students require foundational courses before they are able to be successful in this kind of coursework. However, let's consider that 55% of nurses hold a bachelor's degree (DiMattio & Spegman, 2019), 13% have graduate degrees, and less than 1% have doctoral degrees (AACN, 2019). Most nurses who work at the bedside are not educated to be empowered change agents, and those with advanced degrees are expected to be change agents. This education culture sends a clear message to bedside nurses— changing the system is not their problem.

Finally, higher education is less about teaching information and more about teaching a person how to think and solve problems. Nursing education is hyper-focused on preparing students to pass the NCLEX®. Passing the NCLEX exam is important as academic programs are rated based on pass rates and they may lose accreditation if their rates drop below a certain rate. It is understandable that programs teach to the test. Is passing a test the only reliable measure of a school's success? In addition to NCLEX pass rates, shouldn't a nursing school be able to proudly promote rates of their students going on to become nurse entrepreneurs, inventors, and change agents?

In order to have real systemic impact, nurses must be taught to be change agents beyond the bedside. This begins by educating and empowering all nurses to be change agents within the healthcare system and beyond. Imagine a potential student shopping for a nursing program and finding a brochure that ensures they'll pass the NCLEX as well as be prepared to change the world. We will come back to this vision at the end of this chapter.

Nursing Science and Academia

My PhD program interview was a disaster. At some point in my interview, the professor who was interviewing me asked, "Why do you want to get a PhD?" I responded, confidently, "I want to be a scientist. I want to do high impact research. I do not want to do any of the fluffy nursing studies I read about in nursing school. You know the ones—how do patients feel after a vasectomy revision? Yeah, I don't want to do any of that, ever. I want to do work that really helps people."

Yes, I said all of that in an interview. What I didn't know was that I was talking to a nationally recognized and respected qualitative researcher; and everything I said was an insult to her work. Fortunately for me, she liked me well enough and realized I had no idea I was insulting her preferred method—qualitative research. I was admitted to the program. Ironically, after 5.5 years of study, I defended my qualitative dissertation study with the professor I insulted in my initial interview serving as one of my mentors and a key member of my dissertation committee.

In retrospect, I realize that it was all of the experiences in nursing programs and with academic nurses that led me to form some very strong opinions about nursing "science and research." Though misguided, and aside from my display of blatant ignorance, my opinions on nursing academics were not completely unfounded during my interview.

Up until my interview I had been living in the research-to-practice gap. I was a perpetual student in nursing programs, and I worked continuously as a nurse. I spent years between the juxtaposition of nursing theory and history and the real-life work of a nurse. As a working student nurse, I was often inspired by new knowledge, equally dismayed by learning about things that seemed to not matter at all, and disheartened that the real-world problems I faced as a nurse were almost never addressed in an academic setting. I was living and practicing in the real world of nursing and it seemed that the academic programs were based of a false reality of the world.

Throughout my studies I almost never met an academic nurse who did something meaningful in my lifetime, nor was I taught about any revolutionary contemporary nurses. By the time I made it to my PhD interview, I had worked as a nursing assistant and an LPN; had earned an associate's degree, bachelor's degree, master's degree, and completed NP training; and was teaching nurses. I had worked in many settings and studied at several levels. My opinion of nursing academics was that "they" were all princesses in ivory towers, living the good life, while most nurses toiled in the gutters. It seemed to me that the schools minimally prepared me to go to work, and didn't tell me about the real world. Importantly, it seemed there was no bridge between the two worlds of academia and practice, and I wanted to make one.

Academic-to-Self-Advocacy Gap

Academic nurses have discussed the theory-to-practice gap ad nauseam. Greenway, Butt, and Walthall define the gap this way:

> The gap between the theoretical knowledge and the practical application of nursing, most often expressed as a negative entity, with adverse consequences. (2019, p. 1)

While the idea of a theory-to-practice gap is a real problem regarding the application of nursing science, a similar problem exists in the gap between nursing practice and self-advocacy. I would describe this as a practice-to-self-advocacy gap, and define it as the gap between learned or experienced nursing practice and self-advocacy as a culture and practice.

Much like the theory-to-practice gap, the practice-to-self-advocacy gap has adverse consequences. For example, a 2019 study found that one-third of new graduate nurses leave the bedside within the first 2 years of practice (AACN, 2019). There may be several reasons why this phenomenon is happening, including difficult practice settings, understaffing, and the increasing draw to seek advanced practice. Regardless, if one-third of new graduate nurses entering the workforce plan to leave the practice setting with the greatest need, we have failed to prepare them in some way.

We prepare nursing graduates to pass the NCLEX and give them all of the basic skills to "do the job." However, we do not educate them on the realities of nursing in modern healthcare, and we certainly do not prepare them with enough skills and knowledge to actually "do something" to change the systems that are driving them from the bedside.

Publish or Perish

Nursing academics isn't immune from the "publish or perish" culture of higher education. However, to speak candidly, practicing bedside nurses are not very interested in these studies. They don't read them and even if they are interested in reading them, the studies are often so convoluted and the results so ambiguous that they're less than helpful. Nurses are interested in any promising and practical solutions that improve efficiencies, reduce redundancy, improve safety, and make their work more manageable.

Nurse scientists, the most educated of the nurses, are often bogged down with trying to create new knowledge in order to get tenure or remain relevant in their fields. Moreover, these nurses are often so removed from the bedside that their perception of the realities of nursing is skewed. Despite my attempts not to become distanced from the bedside, as a PhD student I found myself far removed from the typical nurse view. Still, I did what all budding academics do—I buckled down and completed my program with hopes of returning to more meaningful and impactful work in the future.

In my first year in graduate school to become an NP, our class was invited to attend a summit. The keynote speaker was a renowned nursing theorist from Boston.

In her talk, the speaker discussed her vision for the future of nursing, with the DNP degree being the entry-way to practice. In other words, the starting degree for the professional nurses would be a doctorate.

In typical fashion, I had not reviewed who this theorist was, nor the importance of her work. I had no idea who I was sharing the room with and didn't know I was sitting in a room full of scholars and academics, with PhDs and decades of experience behind them. I didn't think twice to ask a simple question and was the first person to be recognized when she opened the floor for questions.

I prefaced the question as follows:

"We've only recently agreed that the bachelor's degree would be the starting degree. We have staffing shortages all around the country, and not enough nurses to replace the retiring ones. Do you actually believe that a person would or should get a doctoral degree and then be willing to work a night shift in a nursing home, and is that a realistic or feasible expectation?"

The theorist, being an eloquent and experienced orator and scientist, responded, "That was a great question." She then turned the question back to the audience for their opinions.

No one in the crowd could answer the question in a substantive way. The crowd wasn't exactly stumped. It wasn't that the idea of a doctorate being the entry to practice was absolutely ridiculous, as much as it was that the idea was so far removed from the realities of the nursing profession and practice. The fact that she didn't answer my question left me more perplexed than inspired. I was more turned off than interested. More and more I was disheartened and disinterested in what I was getting myself into with the graduate school experience.

The lessons from this interaction were many. First, always know who you are in the room with. This is a lesson I have needed to learn many times over the years. The second, and more important, lesson is that there is, and has been, a huge gap between the creators of science and the people who practice. In the end, I concluded that the theorist from Boston was onto something in that the DNP degree may help bridge this research-to-practice gap to some degree. However, most nurses who receive this kind of doctoral training are not practicing at the bedside with the majority of practicing nurses. So, it was also an impractical solution. If we want to continue elevating nursing as a profession, we should be equally as bold as we are practical, if nothing else.

As scientists we imagine our work to be extremely important. You'll be hard pressed to find a nursing academic, or any academic for that matter, who doesn't dream of discovering something revolutionary. This quest leads us on a chase for the undiscovered. Meanwhile, the challenges we face in healthcare and in nursing are dismissed as low hanging fruit.

When I was studying for my doctorate I wanted to study something that was meaningful and had impact. I worked at a clinic with a predominantly Hispanic population, and our diabetes management outcomes were suboptimal. We also had many patients who were legally disabled, though it was common that the patients and the providers didn't know exactly why they were disabled. Some people were deemed disabled for their entire adult lives. The medical director, my boss at the time, suggested that I study the disability culture in our underserved population of patients. This problem was poorly understood in his opinion. He even offered to help me get access to the data. As a budding scientist, I dismissed this idea as boring. I wanted to go for the gusto. After all, I was becoming a doctor, so I felt I needed to do something bigger and more important. The National Institutes of Health (NIH) was funding studies of diabetes as well as studies of minority populations. Several top schools had great programs that would allow me to continue my research. I chose to study cultural influences on self-care and Puerto Rican adults with diabetes.

Taking on either problem would have been suitable for a doctoral study. However, I believe this kind of thinking is where we go wrong at times. We should think big and dream up new ideas and ways to solve problems; however, we should also think small and common. Thinking small and common may not win us a Nobel Peace Prize, but we're more likely to get the attention of bedside nurses if we are tackling problems they struggle with daily, rather than finding new ones.

Cultish Environment

A nursing faculty shortage looms over the nursing profession. Contributing factors include an aging workforce, low wages, cost of advanced degrees (often required), and emerging career paths (Williamson, 2019). These are not new problems. The elephant in the room is the cultish nursing environment in nursing academics.

Top tier, research-intensive nursing programs are highly selective of their applicants. These programs only take the crème of the crop from large pools of applicants. Nursing programs focused on teaching are also riddled with dysfunction and cattiness that would dismay the most well-intentioned educator. The pay in "lower" tiered programs is often so low that the new graduates easily earn a higher salary than their professors when they enter the workforce with an entry-level nursing position.

A nurse with a doctorate, especially a PhD, is relatively rare. These nurses are expert scientists and clinicians. Despite this expertise and scarcity, these nurses enter academia at the bottom of the totem pole. They must produce new science for approximately 5 years before they're eligible for promotion on the tenure track. They must then continue to produce new science for another 3 to 5 years before they are eligible for a promotion to a tenure track position. As a full professor, they'll earn the salary of a novice NP or an experienced nurse working in a specialty area.

This system takes the "best and brightest" of us, reduces their rank, diminishes their impact, removes them from their peers, and makes it nearly impossible to be connected to the boots on the ground in the profession. In the end, our contemporary nursing scholars don't know nurses and nurses don't know the contemporary scholars.

Nurse Educator Shortage

The nursing profession is facing a shortage of educators. The career path is arduous, and the pay is low compared to that of bedside nurses. Furthermore, some would argue that there are more rewarding career paths for those with graduate education.

Pay Gaps

Nursing education can be divided into three categories: didactic (classroom), clinical, and continuing education. I was thrilled and honored the first time I was asked to be a clinical preceptor. I was equally excited when I had the opportunity to teach didactic courses. However, when the opportunity came to start the job search for full-time faculty positions, I hesitated, and ultimately decided I couldn't afford to leave clinical work to teach. As an experienced NP, the pay cut to work as a nursing faculty would have been $50,000 to $60,000/year. This is the conundrum many nurses with advanced degrees face.

The average nursing faculty earns $74,848 (*Nurse Journal*, 2021), and the average salary for an RN in the United States is $75,510 (U.S. Bureau of Labor Statistics, 2019). Bedside nurses are typically paid hourly and have the potential to earn more if they choose to work extra shifts. Nursing faculty are typically salaried employees. The pay gap between bedside nurses and nursing faculty leaves little incentive for a nurse to become an educator aside from the love of teaching.

Preceptor Shortage

I once worked at a large outpatient clinic where internal medicine residents trained. Every year 20 new interns would join the program, and attending physicians and senior residents would teach them in the clinic.

The model was typical, in that interns and residents would be assigned to an attending physician. They would then conduct exams and formulate plans. As their experience grew, they would be given more autonomy in their practice. The attending physicians' job was to oversee everything they did, ensure that they were learning, and verify that their practice was safe. The attending physicians would sit in a central location while the interns and residents met with the patients. Depending on the experience of the resident, the attending physician would examine or reexamine the patient and revise the plan if needed. The attending physicians' job was to be 100% available to teach their students.

Many student nurses and NP students also trained and completed their clinical rotations at this clinic. Nursing students were paired with a nurse who would assign them tasks and teach them while doing her regular duties. NP students were paired with NP preceptors who had full panels of patients scheduled.

These clinical education models may have varied slightly from institution to institution but were fairly typical. The greatest difference between the physicians and nurses was that the physicians were paid to teach. They were afforded the time and mental space to dedicate their energy to their students, while the nurse preceptors were charged with completing their own work as well as teaching.

Unlike physicians, nurse preceptors are physically burdened by providing clinical education as they are doing two jobs at once. More importantly, while physician educators are paid to precept, nurse preceptors are not paid or compensated at all in any way. It isn't difficult to understand why nursing doesn't have enough clinical educators. There are very few nurses who want to work twice as hard for the same pay.

Lateral Violence

Nursing schools, hospitals, and healthcare institutions in general are often brewing with cattiness and infighting. We even see this being played out on a larger scale with nursing organizations and unions battling over turf, members, and recognition for doing good work. While there are institutions that have a more positive culture, they are relatively rare. Regardless of why we have this culture, where it came from, or why it persists, it must stop if nurses are to become powerful change agents in healthcare.

Lateral violence, or bullying, in nursing starts in nursing education. Faculty bully each other and bully students, students bully each other, preceptors bully students, experienced nurses bully inexperienced nurses, young nurses bully older nurses, and senior nurses bully new nurses. While there has been much discussion in the literature about the phenomena of lateral violence in nursing, the culture remains.

With a bullying culture so pervasive and entrenched, we must actively combat it. It is not enough to simply be a better person as an individual or be the person who does not engage in the negativity. I liken this to racism and bigotry. In order for the culture of racism and bigotry within the United States to change, it wasn't enough for individuals to not be overtly racist. It took an active systemic multilateral push to change the societal norm. To change an interdisciplinary norm of hostility toward each other, it will take all of us actively working to change that culture.

One of the nursing colleges I attended issued a zero-tolerance bullying policy. This policy essentially described consequences for bullying. Still, bullying persisted at every level, especially including faculty and students. The policy outlined how a student or faculty member who was bullied could report the behavior. The problem was that the policy in itself was passive and did not counter the culture of bullying, which was entrenched and prevalent in the school.

Faculty who bully students instill and normalize these behaviors. Those students go on to perpetuate the same behaviors toward each other in their programs and ultimately in their professional roles. This is why a "zero tolerance policy" will not and does not stop the lateral violence phenomenon.

While the idea of "just a nurse" has deeper roots and reaches beyond the educational setting, the remedy begins in education. This is where we begin the healing from within. The education of new nurses is where we begin the conversation that every nurse, regardless of their level of practice or practice setting, is valuable. This is where we teach that the value of a nursing assistant is equal to an RN titrating a dobutamine drip. In order to do this, we must teach all nurses to be change agents and that all nursing roles are valuable.

In the beginning of this chapter we cover some trouble spots in nursing culture. They include the practice of "weeding out the weak ones," hierarchical practice levels undermining unity, pushing the best and brightest away from practice, treating educators poorly, and reinforcing lateral violence in education environments. In the next section let's discuss some practical solutions to these problems.

Academic: Organization

Colleges and schools have the fortunate responsibility and are positioned to rewrite the narrative of negativity in the nursing profession. These institutions can and should do more than prepare nursing students to pass the NCLEX.

Specifically, these schools should redefine the network of nurses, actively combat lateral violence, and use their influence to empower nurses beyond the bedside.

The first and most important thing nursing schools can do to empower their students beyond the bedside is educate them in terms of specific issues affecting the nursing profession. Nursing schools that do this will effectively move all of their students from level 1 to level 2 of engagement.

Nearly all nursing students are taught some version of nursing history. While there is merit in this practice, the history of how Florence Nightingale, and others of her time, founded modern nursing does very little to inspire the next generation of nurses. Nightingale, a scientist and revolutionary thinker, would surely want us to have some modern heroes in the profession. As educators, we should bring this conversation about legacy and professional pride forward and discuss contemporary nursing heroes. The nursing profession is brimming with inspiring contemporary nurses. For example, the story of Nightingale saving lives by instituting handwashing is revolutionary when considering the sanitation standards of her time. However, the story of how the nurses of California were able to organize themselves, campaign, and successfully get a nurse-to-patient ratio bill passed has much more relevance for the everyday nurse. Importantly, the story of that legislative battle can inspire nurses to think of their collective influence beyond the bedside.

Second, nursing schools should create a culture that ensures that the highly educated and/or highly experienced nurses are accessible as resources for nurse innovators, entrepreneurs, and advocates. This means ensuring novice nurses and those at the doctorate level have access to each other. Importantly, it ensures that new nurses are inspired and very experienced and educated nurses have muses for creativity. Simply put, as a profession we need to bring the academics, theorists, and scholars down from the ivory towers and back into the fold of the practice environments. We need these experts to work on the real problems that nurses are experiencing every day. We need these experts to interact on the ground with nurses and to use this collective power, wisdom, and experience to change the healthcare system at the practice and policy level.

Also on this point, nursing schools should address the theory-to-practice gap by educating nurses regarding the gap between academic learning and the realities of practice. Additionally, nursing schools should teach nursing students self-advocacy and nurse innovation as well as introduce them to contemporary nurse entrepreneurs, leaders, and change agents. In doing so, nursing schools will address the practice-to-self-advocacy gap directly.

Third, the nursing profession should place more value on educators. This means paying faculty what they are worth. There is a common idea that people do not become educators or academics out of pursuit of money. However, it is bizarre that in the midst of a nursing faculty shortage, potential faculty candidates are being asked to take a pay cut as they cannot afford to teach full time without working a second clinical job.

Nursing education should be structured similar to residency programs in other disciplines. For example, nurses should be paid to teach students clinically. Furthermore, the clinical environment should allow the educator to focus 100% of their time and effort on their students.

Not all educators are created equal. Passing the NCLEX and having some clinical experience is a very low bar for a clinical educator. Nursing schools should invest in preceptors and clinical educators by teaching them how to teach. Preparing nurses and paying a higher wage may encourage more nurses to precept.

Last, nursing schools should aim to empower the next generation of healthcare change agents who are willing and able to lead healthcare beyond the bedside. The lateral violence culture imbedded in nursing is counterproductive to this aim.

Nursing colleges have the opportunity to counteract lateral violence by creating a counterculture to the phenomenon. This counterculture should emphasize the same kind of unity and comradery present in law enforcement and the military. In addition to teaching clinical skill, nursing schools should instill professional collective ideals in their students. Nursing schools should teach students to support every nurse, regardless of their level of practice, clinical setting, level of education, or geographic location. Novice nurses should enter the workforce with a sense of fraternity.

Nursing faculty should not only be intolerant of lateral violence and bullying; they must also exemplify professional unity. Forward thinking nurse faculty leaders should leave no room for those faculty who cannot adopt this standard. There will surely be resistance to this way of thinking. However, in order to reverse such a powerful negative force embedded in the nursing profession, a drastic approach is required.

Nursing schools should actively combat lateral violence. Instilling comradery shouldn't be limited to nursing students, but should also include preceptorships and mentorships. Nursing culture must shift away from viewing nursing students and new graduate nurses as "baby nurses" and move toward viewing them as allies. Unfortunately, some people may get some tiny satisfaction from looking down on the novice nurse or student. At a systemic level, these behaviors simply create another generation of "mean girls." Changing this deep-rooted culture of lateral violence is not an impossible goal. Consider the unifying culture of law enforcement with the "thin blue line," or the culture within the military, where veterans and active-duty members have a mutual respect for each other.

Making this culture change is not about being "nice," nor is it something we can afford to delay or wait for the next generation to adopt. Lateral violence is an underlying malignancy causing many of the symptoms that plague our profession; we must cut it out before it kills us. This is the kind of culture change the nursing profession needs, and it must begin in nursing education.

Individual Educators

As didactic educators, the impressions we make on nursing students, both positive and negative, are powerful and lasting. If during our student encounters, we do not empower learners clinically and professionally, we have failed them. To empower clinically is to give enough autonomy to boost confidence while guiding safely through the learning process. To empower professionally is to invest in their understanding of the nursing profession and provide them with opportunities to grow beyond the skills of nursing work. As didactic educators, it is our duty to groom nursing students in both ways.

Clinical educators also leave heavy impressions on students and novice nurses. We teach them skill, but we also teach them how to treat each other. Importantly, we teach them how to treat students and novice nurses. As educators, we must be very careful about how we use the relatively short amount of time we spend teaching, and what we may teach subconsciously. Nurses who "eat their young" are doing a great disservice to the learner. More important, they infect the learner with callousness, molding them into the type of clinician who undermines nursing unity and the ability for nurses to organize collectively. If for some reason a nurse clinical educator cannot empower, coach, and groom a learner without belittling them or injuring their spirit, they should excuse themselves from teaching until they acquire enough skill to teach well.

Clinical preceptors are extremely important for the development and education of new nurses as well as novice nurses. However, the role is often thankless and conducted under duress. Many nurses precept students because they themselves were once a student who needed a preceptor. This idea of "owing" the profession some of our time or giving back has terrible consequences. Many nurses simply don't buy into this idea anymore and don't want to precept students. The preceptor shortage is severe enough in some instances that nurses seek clinical training across state lines and are willing to relocate to gain enough hours. Some nursing schools have given up on trying to find clinical preceptors and pawn this responsibility off on the students.

Indeed, we are making the preceptor shortage worse by not taking care of and valuing the clinical educators. Preceptors should demand more from nursing schools in terms of compensation, education, and time. Part of the reason nursing schools don't pay preceptors is the schools are eventually able to convince some nurses to do the work for free. If enough preceptors demanded compensation, the schools would pay. Funding, in this case, is a nonissue. Schools can afford to pay people to teach; even if they couldn't, a "preceptor fee" could be rolled into tuition. There is no real excuse for not compensating professionals for their time or convincing them it is somehow part of their professional duty.

Preceptors should also demand education and training. A good nursing school should invest in vetting their teachers for fit and/or at least teach preceptors "how to teach." Students should be leery of a nursing program with low standards for clinical educators.

Last, preceptors should demand more time. Those precepting for undergraduate nursing programs should not accept teaching assignments while caring for full patient loads. Nurses precepting for graduate programs should demand schedules more in line with nurse residencies where preceptors are paid to teach. The fact that this isn't common practice isn't an issue of lack of funding. I briefly precepted physician assistant students. The school paid the institution where I worked $10,000 per quarter as compensation, and some of those funds were passed directly to preceptors. So the funding is available. When nursing schools avoid paying preceptors, it is not a funding problem. The problem is not enough clinical preceptors have collectively pushed back against the status quo and demanded better.

CONCLUSION

In this chapter we discussed the overall problems and assumptions related to hierarchical learning models. Additionally, we covered several topics within nursing education and academia, including science-to-advocacy gaps, cultish academic environments, the nurse educator shortage, and the ever destructive problem of lateral violence. Finally, we discussed the opportunities for individual nursing professionals and individual educators and opportunities within nursing educational institutions to reform the structures, culture, and behaviors that contribute to the dysfunction within nursing education. Individuals and institutions should aim to adopt and reflect these kinds of changes back onto each individual learner and each academic institution, thereby empowering, unifying, and strengthening the nursing profession and healthcare at large.

DISCUSSION AND REFLECTION POINTS

Hierarchical Learning

1. Reflect on your current role and education level.
2. What motivated you to seek this level of practice?
3. What are your thoughts about nurses practicing with more or less education than you have?
4. What are your thoughts about incorporating training for nurses to be change agents beyond the bedside in nursing curriculum?

Nursing Science and Academia

5. How do you propose decreasing the theory-to-practice gap?
6. How do you propose decreasing the academic-to-self-advocacy gap?
7. What are some practical ways you can inspire and be inspired by bedside nurses in their journey of self-advocacy beyond the bedside?
8. Who are some contemporary nurse innovators, change agents, and entrepreneurs who inspire you?
9. Who are some contemporary nurse scholars who inspire you?
10. What can you do to promote their efforts?

Nurse Educator Shortage

1. What are some barriers to increasing faculty pay?
2. What are some barriers to changing the current unpaid preceptor system?
3. What are the pathways with which you can address these issues within your institution?
4. What are the barriers preventing you from addressing these issues at your institution?

Lateral Violence

1. Have you experienced lateral violence as an educator or student?
2. Were there any pathways for you to address these problems? If so, were they effective?
3. What are some steps you can take right now to ensure the culture of lateral violence stops?

REFERENCES

American Association of Colleges of Nursing. (2019). *The impact of education on nursing practice*. https://www.aacnnursing.org/news-information/fact-sheets/impact-of-education

DiMattio, M. J. K., & Spegman, A. M. (2019). Educational preparation and nurse turnover intention from the hospital bedside. *Online Journal of Issues in Nursing*, 24(2). http://ojin.nursingworld.org/MainMenuCategories/ANAMarketplace/ANAPeriodicals/OJIN/TableofContents/Vol-24-2019/No2-May-2019/Articles-Previous-Topics/Educational-Preparation-and-Nurse-Turnover.html

Greenway, K., Butt, G., & Walthall, H. (2019). What is a theory-gap? An exploration of the concept. *Nurse Education in Practice*, 34, 1–6. https://doi.org/10.1016/j.nepr.2018.10.005

NurseJournal. (2021). *Nursing educator careers and salary outlook*. https://nursejournal.org/careers/nurse-educator

U.S. Bureau of Labor Statistics. (2019). *Occupational employment and wages, May 2018: 29-1141 registered nurses*. https://www.bls.gov/oes/2018/may/oes291141.htm

Williamson, E. (2019). *The nursing faculty shortage problem hasn't gone away*. https://mediakit.nurse.com/nursing-faculty-shortage-problem-gone-away/

4

Fundamental Flaws in the U.S. Healthcare Model

INTRODUCTION

Most nurses are well acquainted with their work and related duties. As a rule, nurses are generally diligent and dedicated to the care they give their patients. Unfortunately, caring for a patient, or many patients, offers a narrow view into the healthcare industry, what entities control the industry, and how to access the people within those entities. This chapter is a discussion about who controls healthcare, how nurses fit into the model, and small and large steps every nurse can take to take more control of the system.

Discovering the Model

I once attended a talk by renowned nursing theorist Dr. Jacqueline Fawcett, in which she described her vision of the future of nursing. Her pitch was a future that included "nursing facilities." These facilities would be managed and staffed entirely by nurses, who would also provide nursing care. At the time, I was a PhD student, and turned my nose up at the idea. I asked myself, why on earth do we need "nursing" hospitals? It would take years before I truly understood the wisdom of Dr. Fawcett's vision. My deduction from her vision—the current system doesn't support or value the work of nursing; therefore, nurses need to own and manage their own facilities.

Throughout my professional years, I practiced in various levels of nursing. I also worked in a variety of settings. One thing that was constant throughout all of my experiences was the way I was treated as a nurse. In many respects I was valuable, useful, and essential for my patients and colleagues. My employers also treated me as an expensive cog in a wheel, something to be managed and to be squeezed until I was at the limits of my productivity.

I noticed that nurses who were sitting down and not actively doing something were viewed and treated as a cost to their employer. Highly skilled human beings who provided intangible service and care were treated no differently than a light bulb or a mop head. This way of treating nurses plays out in many ways. On the one hand, nurses are burned out very easily because they're pushed to the limits as employers try to get the most for their money. On the other hand, employers are constantly looking for ways to get the services of nursing without paying a nurse wage.

For instance, over the past decades we've seen a push from long-term care facilities lobbying to allow med techs (nursing assistants) to administer medications under the "remote supervision of a nurse."

I have worked as a nurse's aide. Nursing assistants are skilled and talented and add immeasurable value to the healthcare system. Nearly anyone can be trained to pass a pill to a person. However, a nurse assistant is not trained to administer medications with the breadth and depth of knowledge that a nurse has. For example, nurse assistants are not trained to monitor for side effects, check for interactions, and so on. Nursing assistants are, however, much cheaper than a licensed nurse. As we move through this chapter, remember this point: The goal of the employer is to make a profit; all of the services in healthcare are merely by-products of attempting to create profit for the institution and its shareholders. These are not necessarily negative aspects of the healthcare industry, but rather facts we must understand if we aim to improve the system.

When I started working as a nurse practitioner, my role changed in that I had a foot in the medical camp and a foot in the nursing camp. While my training was as a nurse or APRN, to speak frankly, once licensed I began practicing medicine. My role differed from bedside nursing in that practicing medicine is the diagnosis, treatment, and management of illness. Stepping into this world also meant I generated revenue for my employer. That alone was the single factor in how I was treated differently. This is not to say that I was less busy. I was just as busy as I ever was when I worked as a nurse. However, if I was resting for a moment, taking a break, or for some reason was not actively visiting with my patients, my employer treated me a bit differently. There were still extremely heavy, top–down pressures to perform as well as measurable goals I had to meet in terms of productivity. Burnout was still a very real thing that happened. However, the pressures were indirect. I was asked to see more patients. I was asked to document in more places in the electronic record. I was given less time to get my work done. Indeed, much of the pressure was self-imposed.

The biggest difference I noticed was that there was no overt culture trying to burn me out. I had more vacation time than I'd ever had in my career. There was a cultural norm of taking a short vacation every few months. I was paid more. At times I did feel like a cog in the wheel of a giant machine, but I also felt valued differently. This was largely because I knew that I generated revenue for the organization. My employer in turn treated me like an asset and not a liability. In the business of healthcare, the real difference between nursing practice and medical practice is that medical practice (generally) generates revenue for the organization, while nursing care is considered a cost.

Model Overview

Reimbursement

Money drives everything in healthcare. Our healthcare institutions rely on reimbursement for services they provide. In most cases, outcomes and metrics are used to determine the quality of care, which is driven by reimbursement and to attract more patients. More patients lead to more services, and more services lead to more reimbursement, and so on and so forth. There are three major ways healthcare institutions collect reimbursement for services: Medicare/Medicaid, private health insurance, and private pay (cash). Most senior citizens as well as low-income children and families rely on public health insurance (Medicare and Medicaid) programs as a primary source of healthcare coverage.

Medicare

Medicare is a national health insurance program in the United States, established in 1966, that is managed by the Centers for Medicare and Medicaid Services. Americans over age 65 and some younger people with certain disabilities are eligible for this health insurance. People receiving Medicare benefits may also use private health insurance to supplement any healthcare cost not covered by Medicare. Medicare is financed through a combination of payroll taxes, premiums paid by enrollees, and other subsidies.

Medicare has four parts that cover various healthcare costs. Part A covers inpatient hospital services, Part B covers outpatient services, Part C allows patients to choose equivalent health plans, and Part D covers prescription drugs.

Part A Reimbursement

Reimbursement to a healthcare institution is allocated in the form of a set amount of money for each episode of care provided. This reimbursement is primarily for physician-related services. If the physician services are less than the cost of care, the hospital gets to keep the excess funds. However, if the care exceeds the cost of care, the hospital must cover the costs.

Ideally, a hospital attempts to provide care while minimizing overhead or nonbillable services and resources. In doing so, the hospital can keep more of the reimbursement from health insurance. For example, light bulbs are essential in a hospital that operates 24 hours a day. The hospital may partner with a light bulb manufacturer who can provide long-lasting light bulbs that emit sufficient light and are inexpensive to install, replace, and maintain. If the light bulbs are working well for the hospital, the cost of the light bulbs will not eat into the reimbursement from services the hospital provides. The hospital leadership values the light the bulbs produce and the fact that operations continue throughout the night. However, when a light bulb breaks or stops functioning, it is simply thrown away. It has completed its life cycle. The people who manage the bottom line at the hospital feel no real loss aside from the inconvenience and minor cost of replacing the bulb. The light bulb is a line item.

Nurses, like the light bulb in a hospital, are essential for the hospital to function; however, they do not create revenue through billable services. In an inpatient hospital, the nurse (and illumination from light bulbs) comes with the bed. A hospital may proclaim that they value their nurses; however, they consider bedside nurses as line items. This is because bedside nurses, excluding APRNs, typically do not bill for their services. The people charged with managing hospitals literally place nurses in the same category as light bulbs, secretaries, mop heads, and trash cans—line item costs to be minimized and managed.

Medicaid

Medicaid was established in 1965 and serves as a government insurance program for qualifying low-income Americans. Medicaid eligibility is complex, varies from state to state, and is linked to a person's eligibility to receive Aid to Families With Dependent Children. Funding for Medicaid comes from federal and state-level funding. Reimbursement rates for Medicaid are significantly lower than those for Medicare.

While coverage and rates vary from state to state, Medicaid does cover nursing home care. Again, reimbursement rates are generally very low. For the most part, Medicare does not cover extended nursing home care. (Medicare Part A covers some skilled nursing under certain circumstances.)

Low Medicaid reimbursement rates are devastating to long-term care facilities. These facilities operate similar to inpatient hospitals in that their aim is to minimize the cost of providing care in an attempt to make a profit from the service. Again, nursing staff are treated as line items. This is why the nurse-to-patient ratios in long-term care are unfathomable, sometimes exceeding 40 chronically ill geriatric patients to 1 nurse. Nurse salaries are not reflective of their workloads in long-term care and are generally lower than for nurses in inpatient hospital settings. Burnout, high turnover rates, and poor patient care are rampant and common in many long-term care facilities. This is all related to long-term care facilities attempting to use the least amount of "resources"—that is, nurses—available and bag a small profit from the miniscule reimbursement system.

Private Insurance

Private insurance is the primary source of coverage for most people (61%) in the United States (Cohen et al., 2020). While medical care has existed for hundreds of years, health insurance has only existed in the United States for approximately 170 years and employer group health insurance for only 110 years. Prior to these payment options, patients used a fee-for-service option and would pay out of pocket for the services or care they received. In this scheme, patients and/or employers pay premiums, and in most cases the health insurance company covers the cost of routine, preventive, and emergency healthcare services as well as the cost of prescription and over-the-counter drugs. Health insurance companies use a formulary (a prefabricated list) to decide what types of healthcare services (drugs, test, etc.) they cover. Services not included on this list usually require prior authorization. This prior authorization process was designed with the intent of increasing safety and reducing cost.

Over the past 30 years, health maintenance organizations (HMOs) have soared in popularity; they now represent the majority of employer-based healthcare coverage. An

HMO is a health insurance group that uses managed care to organize and act as a liaison between health insurance and doctors/hospitals. Managed care is/was designed with the intention of reducing healthcare cost and improving quality by only covering certain medical providers and facilities in a "network," focusing on utilization review programs and focusing on primary care. An HMO covers the cost of care by medical providers in their network, and the medical providers in the network benefit by having a steady stream of patients. The utilization management requirement is especially important. This HMO requirement is meant to assure quality and requires accreditation in order to receive reimbursement for healthcare services.

Accreditation

Hospital accreditation is mostly a voluntary process with outcomes tied directly to Medicare reimbursement. There are a few accrediting bodies; The Joint Commission is the most common. These institutions evaluate, provide accreditation, and decide if hospitals can receive reimbursement from Medicare.

Hospitals that rely on Medicare reimbursement must comply with The Joint Commission standards. The Joint Commission reports that their board of commissioners includes

> 21 voting members, including physicians, administrators, nurses, employers, quality and innovation experts, and educators. The Board includes representatives from each of the Joint Commission's Corporate Members: American Hospital Association, American Medical Association, American College of Physicians, American College of Surgeons, and American Dental Association. (The Joint Commission, n.d., "Board Facts")

Corporate members like the American Hospital Association and American Medical Association have outright lobbying arms and very deep pockets. Importantly, many of the board members are executives at, or work closely with, the large health systems The Joint Commission oversees. All of this information is available to the general public (The Joint Commission, n.d.).

Who Controls Healthcare?

The healthcare industry is nearly self-regulated and unchecked in many ways. Throughout my career I've complained, and heard other healthcare workers complain, about the inadequacies of the system. Often, the complaints and frustration are directed toward mid-level managers (charge nurses, unit managers, medical directors, etc.). Some broad thinkers directed me further up the line, implicating hospital CEOs and owners. This is a plausible direction to focus frustration as healthcare has become top heavy with many moving parts unrelated to direct patient care. Some "[e]stimates suggest that between 15–30 percent of overall health care spending, and one-quarter of the medical labor force, are involved in costs of billing, insurance management, hospital administration, and the like" (Gottlieb & Shepard, 2018, "The Facts").

Understandably, with overinflated salaries of hospital administrators, and a plethora of nonclinical employees roaming around healthcare facilities, these people are easy places to target frustrations. They are somewhat visible, not quite accessible, and don't provide the direct care the institution was built to provide. These employees are low hanging fruit and focusing our frustration on them rarely yields any substantive change.

For many years throughout my career I steered my frustration and angst toward nonclinical employees and administrators. When I started working with grassroots nursing groups that were working on staffing legislation, I couldn't understand why such simple solutions were stalled in the legislative process. For example, I couldn't understand why, if most hospital-based nurses believed limits on the number of patients was the best and safest care, only California and a few other states in the union passed laws mandating a limit on nurse-to-patient ratios. This question led me to try and understand who actually controls healthcare and, importantly, how to gain access to the controls.

Here are the facts. The healthcare business model primarily makes profits by collecting reimbursement from health insurance and minimizing cost of care. HMOs require hospitals to be accredited in order to receive reimbursement. Accreditation bodies are managed by individuals and corporate members. These individuals and corporate members of accreditation bodies are connected to the hospital systems the body accredits. Importantly, individuals and corporate members of these accreditation bodies are connected to powerful lobbyists. The job of powerful lobbyists is to influence lawmakers at the local, state, and federal levels.

The contemporary healthcare system is designed to make profit. It is controlled by those who regulate the industry, and the regulators arrange the system to make profit. The point is mid-level hospital managers, or even executives and other healthcare administrators, are near the bottom of the barrel in this scheme. They are not the cause of the problem, but rather a symptom of a systemic problem of how the healthcare system functions. As nurses, we feel these symptoms. We feel undervalued, underrepresented, and ignored. This is because nurses are factored into this equation as a cost, a liability to be managed and minimized.

Contemporary Healthcare and Nursing

Problems and Consequences

Hospitals aren't reimbursed directly for nursing care. For example, the hospital can submit a claim for reimbursement when a medical provider treats an infection with intravenous (IV) antibiotics as well as the supplies used (IV catheter, tubing, medication, etc.). However, the hospital cannot receive reimbursement for the time or effort the nurse used when hanging the fluid or inserting the IV.

The primary consequence of this model is that the hospital must push the nurse to be as productive as possible during the time they are working. To minimize the cost of the nurse, hospital systems assign the "maximum" amount of work possible for each nurse to "safely" complete in a shift. The maximum amount of work a nurse can safely be assigned will vary from shift to shift, unit to unit, hospital to hospital, and health system to health system. However, the way nurses fit into the model is consistent throughout healthcare.

Ultimately, this system by default minimizes the importance of nursing care by equating nursing care with lost revenue. It is no wonder nurses consistently report feeling underrepresented and undervalued. The system was not designed to benefit nurses; it was designed to benefit physicians. This is quite evident as medical provider services (including APRNs) are the core element of the reimbursement scheme between medical providers and health insurers. Physician services are essential within and throughout the healthcare system in the United States. However, physicians cannot manage hospital patients without nurses. In fact, safe operation of a hospital requires significantly more nurses than physicians. That being said, the systemic problems nurses face are not the fault of our individual, highly valued physician colleagues. The fault lies with the accrediting bodies and lobbyists that continue to build on and capitalize from this heavily nurse-reliant but physician-centric system.

Reimbursement Linked to Quality

Working conditions in healthcare facilities are tied to regulatory bodies. Importantly, reimbursement is tied to accreditation, which is tied to quality measures. Quality of patients' care is linked to medical and nursing care. For example, Medicare penalizes hospitals that readmit a patient for the same diagnosis within 30 days of the most recent admission by not reimbursing for the second admission. Treatment for hospital-acquired infections are also not reimbursed. These kinds of well-intentioned policies are designed to improve the quality of care patients receive.

Nurses, and other healthcare providers, in hospital settings are often charged with documenting and recording that quality measures are met. For example, nurses are responsible for changing central line dressings and documenting this work. If a patient develops sepsis related to an infection at their central line entry point, the hospital may not be reimbursed for the complications and treatments needed to care for the patient.

Nurses are linked directly to quality measures and indirectly to reimbursement. This model amplifies the nurse as an asset when performance measures are met and as a liability when they aren't met. This is also why top–down management pressures don't feel like they are patient centric. The manager who harps on the nurses about documentation is literally a cog in the wheel, playing their position and ensuring the hospital doesn't lose revenue. The executives who introduce new documentation procedures are usually trying to satisfy accrediting bodies.

In the trenches, it can feel like these administrators don't care about the staff. This is not the case. Administrators are not inherently evil; they are simply trying to increase revenue and prevent losses to the institution.

The contemporary healthcare model creates chasms between frontline staff and hospital administrators. Consequences include staff muddling through "busy work," often with little understanding of how the tasks are linked to quality measures. Nurses and healthcare providers document defensively as they don't believe the institution understands their work or will back them if a mistake is made. The system encourages administrators to use nurses like pawns to achieve certain outcomes.

For example, low patient satisfaction scoring systems like the Hospital Consumer Assessment of Healthcare Providers and Systems (HCAHPS) survey, also known as H-Caps, can affect hospital reimbursement. HCAHPS measures how patients perceive their care experience. These seemingly well-intentioned tools are intended to shed light on where hospitals can improve their processes and care. Medicare reimbursement is also tied to patient satisfaction surveys like HCAHPS.

Some HCAHPS questions pertaining to nursing care and the hospital environment include the following:

- During this hospital stay, how often did nurses treat you with courtesy and respect?
- During this hospital stay, how often did nurses listen carefully to you?
- During this hospital stay, after you pressed the call button, how often did you get help as soon as you wanted it?
- During this hospital stay, how often was the area around your room quiet at night?
- How often did you get help in getting to the bathroom or in using a bedpan as soon as you wanted?

The criteria for an inpatient hospital admission is complex, but generally mandate that a person requires at least 48 hours of continuous monitoring, care, or testing to diagnose and treat a serious medical or psychiatric condition. The types of questions in HCAHPS reflect the type of service hotel customers would expect. These highly subjective questions about nursing care are factored into Medicare reimbursement and absurdly reflect the idea that a person who is suffering from a serious medical condition should expect to have a good "experience." In the real world of nursing, this can play out as real consequences for patients and staff.

For instance, let's take the example of Patient A, a 50-year-old man being evaluated in the ED for chest pain and cough, and Patient B, a 25-year-old woman being evaluated for nontraumatic wrist pain. Imagine Patient A starts having difficulty breathing and medical staff need to work together to insert a chest tube to save his life. Simultaneously, Patient B has been waiting for several hours in the next room; she would like to request a snack and has pushed the call light several times with the same request. After the chest tube is placed in Patient A's chest, the nurse ensures the patient is safe and then rushes to respond to Patient B's call light. Patient A feels abandoned after his procedure. Patient B feels abandoned after waiting so long to receive food. Both patients give negative scores for nursing services on their HCAHPS surveys.

Now, imagine this situation playing out over and over again. The quality and compliance department notices the low HCAHPS scores and pushes the unit managers to improve the scores. The Joint Commission surveys notice the low HCAHPS scores and flag the hospital with a warning, which ultimately affects reimbursement for services. Now, hospital administrators add additional pressure on unit managers to improve HCAHPS scores. Nurses and medical staff are encouraged to not only save lives but also provide pleasant, cheerful, and prompt service to customers.

In this scenario, the hospital could add more nurses, which would avoid the situation that played out between Patient A and Patient B; however, this would be an additional cost to the hospital. Subsequently, in order to keep up with the standards of quality management and accrediting bodies, the unit managers ask the nurses to do more with less. Nurses are asked to document more, be in multiple places at once, and ensure patients are satisfied customers. Nurses become frustrated with the top–down pressures from the managers. They become frustrated with the inability to produce quality care, while simultaneously producing data to meet accreditation metrics. The nurses' work becomes consumed by documenting defensively. Managers become frustrated with the nurses' inability to produce the needed results to satisfy the accrediting bodies and quality control, and executives become frustrated with the nursing department. This general scenario plays out in hospitals all around the United States year after year and has been an ongoing struggle for decades. In these types of scenarios, nearly all of the nurses are frustrated because the system isn't designed for them to succeed or feel valued.

It's easy to understand why nurses are so frustrated with HCAHPS. Health systems use these metrics and expect nurses to be maids and servants instead of healthcare professionals. They go so far as to reprimand nurses when patients are unhappy with the "service" they receive. This idea of providing customer services instead of care undermines the value of the entire nursing profession.

Reclaiming Control of Healthcare

Targeting the Controls

One of the reasons nurses haven't had success in claiming a substantive voice in healthcare is the culture of focusing professional angst and frustration toward people and entities that cannot and will not change the system to benefit nurses. When a nurse is asked to assume care for an unsafe number of patients, they typically vent, to no avail, frustrations about nursing administrators and/or the healthcare facility. The problem is the system that treats nurses as liabilities is not controlled by nursing administrators or the healthcare facility. The administrator and the healthcare facility subsequently don't make adequate changes to accommodate the nurse. The nurse feels unsupported and eventually burns out.

The first step bedside nurses can take to reclaim power in healthcare is to understand who controls the healthcare system. The ladder of engagement model can be used to ensure that every nurse in the U.S. healthcare system is aware of who controls nursing facilities and is actively asserting their voice to ensure nurses are put in positions that can actually improve the system.

Nurses at level 1 engagement are generally unaware of the problem. These nurses may be students, novices, and/or experienced nurses. Academic institutions should include discussions in the curriculum detailing how the accreditation process functions and how it dictates how the healthcare system works. All graduating nursing students should know and understand where they should direct attention if they wish to improve the system for nurses.

Novice nurses to experienced nurses may not be aware of who controls the healthcare system, or who to hold accountable for improving the system for nurses. All nurses should investigate specifically how their facility makes profit, what accreditation body monitors their facility, and who their nurse representative is who sits on the board of directors within that accrediting institution (if one is present). This board member is the person to whom complaints, frustrations, and suggestions should be sent. A charge nurse has limited control over unsafe staffing; however, a nurse board member of an accrediting body actually helps make rules and guidance that dictate reimbursement for a facility. These individuals are the only people who can effectively influence and/or change how a healthcare facility operates.

Nurses at level 2 are aware of, but not engaged in, addressing the problem, and nurses at level 3 of engagement are minimally engaged in addressing the problem. These nurses may include those who lead nursing associations or organizations. These nurses are likely aware that accrediting bodies control healthcare systems and they may or may not be actively engaging accreditors with the aim of improving and influencing the system. Nurses who belong to nursing associations and organizations should understand how accreditation affects their healthcare institution and know their representative on the board. Additionally, these nurses should demand that their nursing organization engage board members of the accrediting bodies that oversee their institution.

Nurses at levels 4, 5, and 6 are moderately to highly engaged, and/or activists addressing the problem. These nurses may include those high-ranking board members of accrediting bodies, leaders of professional organizations, and independent nurse advocates.

Nurses on boards of accrediting bodies truly understand the business of healthcare and how nurses fit into the system. These nurses are in a position to challenge the system. However, they are moderately engaged because they have access and ability to make change, but they have not. This is evidenced by the fact that most nurses continue to struggle with similar problems throughout the healthcare system despite having nurses serving as board members in accrediting bodies. Leaders of professional organizations are also in a position to engage accrediting bodies directly. These high-profile nurses represent large numbers of nurses and have influence. Additionally, these nurses have the ability to bring the concerns of the bedside nurse directly to nurses and board members of accrediting bodies.

Both leaders of nursing organizations and nurse board members of accrediting organizations must be open and willing to hear the concerns of bedside nurses and willing to offer bold solutions that consider and prioritize the nursing profession.

Challenge the Reimbursement System

Reimbursement drives nearly every part of the healthcare system. The only way for nurses to assume more control and power within the healthcare system is to move the role of the nurse from a line item expense to an asset that generates revenue. The current system places zero value on the work nurses do but penalizes hospitals when nursing work isn't up to standard. Nurses need to become direct contributors to the healthcare system, not indirect consequences within the system. When a nurse is able to charge individuals and their health insurance provider's company for their services, they not only are valued differently in the system but also are valued differently by patients and the general public.

Levels 1 and 2: Understanding Reimbursement

Nurses at level 1 of engagement are generally unaware of the problem, and those at level 2 of engagement are aware of the problem but are minimally engaged in address-ing the problem. These nurses may be students, nov-ices, and/or experienced nurses. Academic institutions should include discussions in their curriculum detailing how reimbursement systems dictate how the healthcare system works as well as how nurses fit into the system. All graduating nursing students should know and under-stand the business of healthcare and how their service fits into the system. Students should graduate with knowl-edge of how the healthcare system places low value on their efforts, whom to contact to advocate for change, and how to advocate to change the system.

Novice nurses to experienced nurses may not be aware of how the reimbursement system in health-care undermines and devalues the nursing profession. These nurses should at the very least seek to under-stand how their healthcare system and facilities profit and receive reimbursement as well as what nursing services or quality measures are tied to reimbursement. All nurses should know what accreditation body moni-tors their facility and who their nurse representative is that sits on the board of directors within that accred-iting institution (if one is present). Finally, all nurses should discuss these issues formally and informally in the workplace, with the aim of ensuring every nurse is aware of the specific ways the healthcare system deval-ues nurses.

Levels 3 and 4: Social Campaigns

Nurses at levels 3 and 4 of engagement are aware of the problem but are minimally to moderately engaged in addressing the problem. For example, these nurses may be minimally to moderately engaged in self nurse advo-cacy. They may advocate for themselves independently, advocate with others, and/or be members of professional organizations. In addition to levels 1 and 2 of engagement, these nurses should find and/or initiate social media campaigns to facilitate interprofessional and extraprofessional dialogue about the healthcare reimbursement system. These campaigns should target leaders of professional organizations and board members of accrediting bodies as well as the general public. The aim of these campaigns should be to generate positive, but disruptive dialogue about how the role of the nurse is undermined by the reimbursement system and advocating for nursing services to be included as a billable service.

Levels 5 and 6: Organizations, Accreditors, Legislators

Nurses at levels 5 and 6 are highly engaged in addressing the problem as activists. These nurses may include leaders of professional organizations, board members of accrediting bodies, and activists focused on addressing the problem of nurses being excluded from the reimbursement system. Leaders of nursing associations, organizations, and unions are aware that nursing services are not reimbursable in the current healthcare system as this has been the status quo and the system they are accustomed to operating within. These nurses may or may not understand that this model ultimately undermines the efforts, power, and control nurses have within the system.

Accrediting bodies control healthcare systems, and the nurses appointed to boards of directors of these accrediting bodies have influential positions. These nurses may or may not be actively engaging their fellow board members with the aim of improving and influencing the role of nurses within the healthcare system. As representatives of the nursing profession, these nurses should use their influence and expertise to empower nurses individually and collectively. These influential nurses should seek out dialogue with their frontline nurse colleagues and use this valuable feedback to guide their decisions in the boardroom.

CONCLUSION

In this chapter we covered healthcare reimbursement, entities that control healthcare, how nurses fit into the healthcare model, and some strategies to help nurses assume more control of the healthcare system. In order for nurses to claim control of the healthcare system, nurses must connect their service to reimbursement as well as interact with and influence the people who control healthcare. Using the ladder of engagement described earlier, every nurse can involve themselves, minimally or exhaustively, in helping nurses have more influence in healthcare. In the next chapter we discuss leadership and empowerment.

DISCUSSION AND REFLECTION POINTS

1. What new information did you learn about the healthcare reimbursement structure?
2. What are some things you can do to help nurses become assets in the healthcare system?
3. What did you learn about the healthcare facility accreditation system?
4. What is the accrediting body for the healthcare facility where you work, train, or receive care?
   a. Is there a nurse board member?
   b. How do you contact this person?

REFERENCES

Cohen, R. A., Cha, A. E., Martinez, M. E., & Terlizzi, E. P. (2020). *Health insurance coverage: Early release of estimates from the National Health Interview Survey*. https://www.cdc.gov/nchs/data/nhis/earlyrelease/insur202009-508.pdf

Gottlieb, J. D., & Shepard, M. (2018). *How large a burden are administrative costs in health care?* https://econofact.org/how-large-a-burden-are-administrative-costs-in-health-care

The Joint Commission. (n.d.). *Board of Commissioners*. https://www.jointcommission.org/en/about-us/facts-about-the-joint-commission/board-of-commissioners

5

Leadership and Empowerment

INTRODUCTION

Every nurse is a leader. The process of completing health-care training, establishing oneself as a human caretaker, and joining a global network of healers establishes a nurse as a leader. The degree to which each nurse leads will vary, but every nurse leads in one way or another. Despite the nurses' natural propensity toward leadership, the COVID-19 pandemic of 2020 illustrated the lack of nursing leadership at every level perfectly.

In this chapter we discuss nursing leadership at the national, institutional, and individual levels; identify the lack of nursing leadership in healthcare; and discuss pathways to increase nurse leadership throughout healthcare. There are books, theories, articles, and oodles of people who give instruction on "leadership" and how to be a "good leader" or even an "excellent leader." Among all of these guides are a plethora of works outlining "nursing leadership" and describing how to be a nurse leader. Yet, as a profession, we find ourselves without substantial leadership within the healthcare system. The elephant in the room is that healthcare is dominated by nurses, yet nurses do not lead healthcare. This conundrum has perplexed me for years.

There are several factors contributing to the lack of nursing leadership in healthcare. These include but are not limited to a history of subordination, professional infighting, and professional shortsightedness. Some of these pitfalls are woven tightly into the culture of professional nursing.

National Leadership

There is no unifying national nursing organization in the United States. This is largely due to the fractured and dysfunctional organizational culture within the nursing profession. Nursing organizations, as a rule, do not work in unison, nor do they agree on their methods of empowering individual nurses and/or the nursing profession. Moreover, most nurses are not members of the largest, self-proclaimed, national nursing organizations.

As national (or international) healthcare-related problems arise, the public does not turn to "national nursing organizations" as a healthcare authority. Moreover, and generally, national nursing organizations are not viewed as authorities on healthcare and due to the fractured member base and messaging do not lead the nursing profession or healthcare at large. To put this in immediate context, during the COVID-19 global pandemic, frontline healthcare providers were understaffed, were under-resourced, and bore the brunt of the virus as healthcare systems became overwhelmed. The problems with understaffing and nurses not having enough protective equipment trended on international news, national news, and social media networks for months. All of the nursing organizations made statements about the issues nurses were facing, and many made efforts to help frontline healthcare workers. Yet none of the major nursing organizations in the United States made the national or international news circuit in any substantial way. The individual efforts of nursing organizations went largely unnoticed. In this instance, professional shortsightedness was on full display. The COVID-19 global pandemic was an opportunity for nursing organizations to unite behind one common cause and elevate the nursing profession as the science-based global leader in healthcare. This did not happen. Truthfully, the world has yet to turn to the nurse for solutions to big healthcare problems.

Institutional Leadership

In Chapter 4, we discussed who controls healthcare and how institutional nursing leaders are often powerless by comparison. The reimbursement system in healthcare ensures that all nursing leaders, from the chief nursing officer to the night shift charge nurse, are empowered just enough to minimize losses associated with employing nurses but not empowered enough to disrupt the system at large. The healthcare system places some nurses in positions of "authority" in such a way that it gives the illusion of authority, yet these nurses are not actually empowered enough to lead their institutions. At best, nurse leaders within institutions can mitigate revenue losses and be buffers between corporate leadership and nursing staff. Again, throughout the COVID-19 pandemic, institutional nursing leadership proved to be relatively powerless when it came to protecting their staff.

Individual Leadership

Nurses truly shine at the individual leadership level. Individual nurses are trusted by the public and by their peers. However, there is a history of subordination imposed by the practice of medicine onto the practice of nursing. Historically, most physicians were men. The practice of nursing was dictated by and delegated from male physicians to female nurses. These demographics are now shifting, with more women becoming physicians and more men becoming nurses. However, the system that positions one group as reliant on and deferential to the other still exists. A classic example of this dynamic is that nurses still rely on "orders" from medical providers to conduct some of their work. This is a long-standing and necessary part of the healthcare system. However, the overtones and subsequent culture this creates undermine nurses leading in healthcare.

Still, the history of nurses being subordinate is an old narrative. In this narrative, women in little white hats stand when a physician enters the room, slink into the background, and retrieve a cup of coffee prepared "just the way he likes it." These days are long gone, but the paradigm still exists to some degree.

Hope is not lost. More and more, we see nurses practicing at the highest level of their licensure, asserting their insights and skills, and working alongside physicians as colleagues and team members. To shift this narrative even further, nurses must remove this concept of subordination from the profession entirely and assume a position of professional parity with physician colleagues. This is not to say that nurses and physicians have the same knowledge base or training but rather the professions are equally reliant on each other to provide care. This bold kind of vision would recognize that both physician and nurse roles are equally important. The modern healthcare system does not allow space for a physician to physically provide care for wards full of patients. The physician is reliant on the nurse to do this work. Similarly, the system is designed in such a way that even very qualified nurses rely on expert medical opinions and direction from physicians. Nurses are not trained physicians and rely on physicians for complex medical decision-making.

CHANGING THE NARRATIVE

The lack of nursing leadership within healthcare is an old narrative. The void of nursing leadership at the national and international levels is a direct result of professional shortsightedness. Leaders of professional nursing organizations are so bogged down in dogmatic approaches and territorial squabbles that they rarely make it to the national or international stage. Nurses at the institutional leadership level are mostly concerned with being a buffer between senior leadership and staff. At the individual level, nurses are mostly concerned with patients and communities.

This professional shortsightedness is a symptom of the history of subordination and professional infighting. Nursing professional culture is such that nurses are satisfied with simply being noticed enough to be invited to the leadership table. This mentality is part of the problem. As the largest force within healthcare, nurses should have significant representation at leadership tables at every level.

Every nurse is a leader in some way. However, for nurses to lead and revolutionize healthcare, every nurse must extend their leadership beyond the bedside. There are three essential principles that will help every nurse lean into their leadership potential: knowing one's preferred leadership style, recognizing and filling systemic voids, and positive disruption to the status quo.

The first and most important factor in leadership is to know and understand what type of leader you are. There are many leadership styles. The information in Box 5.1 is not an exhaustive list of definitions of these leadership styles but rather is meant to highlight the positive attributes of each leadership style. These leadership styles may be useful in healthcare settings.

The most important first step is to recognize and embrace your preferred leadership style. Some would argue that certain leadership styles are better than others. This is misleading. Each leadership style can be useful. To be effective, the style should be comfortable for the leader and appropriate for the situation. For example, in a small group medical practice, where all of the team members are equally competent and ranked, a democratic leadership style may be helpful. Contrarily, in military medicine, an autocratic style may be more useful. Every nurse should spend some time understanding what leadership style suits them.

BOX 5.1 Leadership Type Definitions

Visionary: Inspirational, drive progress, earn trust easily

Servant: Work alongside the team, focus on colleague satisfaction, morale builders

Autocratic: Authoritarian, efficiency and compliance focused

Democratic: Consideration of team input fosters high employee engagement

Transformational: Focus on communication, goals, commitment to organization

Transactional: Focus on mentorship, achieving goals, enjoying rewards

Throughout my career I've been gently pushed into leadership positions. This was likely due to several factors, including being a man, my personality, my work ethic, and having some level of ambition. However, I was never interested in leadership in any way. In fact, I balked at the idea of being "in charge of anyone" aside from myself. This attitude persisted even as I was being nudged into leadership roles while I completed several nursing programs, worked several different kinds of healthcare-related jobs, and was well into my doctoral training.

During my last graduate degree training, the dean of the school mandated leadership training as part of doctoral education, specifically for academic degrees. He gave the rationale that too many people were graduating with PhDs who didn't understand leadership. Nonetheless, it was during this training that I learned that I prefer the servant leadership style. This likely stems from my own discomfort with authority and not wanting to be a "bossy boss." This was a powerful revelation and allowed me to step into leadership roles with more comfort as I knew how I preferred to lead. The revelation was that people sought me out as a leader because I liked to lead from within the pack. This was comfortable for the people who worked with me but also comfortable for me as I didn't even recognize I was enjoying leadership.

The second principle that helps nurses lean into leadership is recognizing and filling systemic voids. Every employed nurse can point out the dysfunction, problems, and issues within the healthcare system or institution in which they work. Recognizing the problems, or the voids, in the system is rarely a problem for nurses. Nurses struggle with taking action to fill the voids they see.

The third factor in leadership is positive disruption of the status quo. Taking bold action can be difficult and downright terrifying, especially if we consider our livelihood is tied to what we do or do not do professionally.

However, in order to really step into leadership, nurses must stop asking for permission to do the right thing. We must be brave enough to do the right thing and challenge those in power to contest us publicly for doing what is right. We should never push ethical or moral boundaries. However, professional boundaries are fair game if our actions are truly making things better.

I worked for a large agency that had high turnover at the medical director level, so much so that there were three new medical directors within 3 years, as well as rapid turnover at the medical provider level. Staff morale was low, and the patients were frustrated with poor care continuity. Word "on the street" was that medical care at this agency was not very good.

The regulatory bodies for this specialty required a physician to serve as medical director and oversee the medical practice at this agency. The agency charged the medical director with overseeing the department in which I worked as well as provided care to patients. This model excluded me, a nurse, from leadership within the agency. However, my time working at the agency allowed me to see the problem differently than senior leadership.

As an APRN I wasn't sure exactly what the medical director job entailed, but I knew there was likely a systemic problem. I knew the agency was far too large and the practice far too unwieldy for one person to manage. I made a proposal to the senior leadership that I take on some of the responsibilities of the medical director role on a trial basis. My compromise was that I would work my regular clinical job in addition to helping at the leadership level.

As a servant leader, this was most suitable for me. I loved to work alongside the providers and solve problems. My goal was to make the agency a destination for nurses and providers. I believed that if we took better care of the staff, they would in turn take better care of the patients.

I worked tirelessly in this unofficial role for 1.5 years, during which time I studied the problems and worked with other staff to fix them. After 12 months of work, the medical department stabilized. After 18 months, the medical department was completely transformed. We hired excellent staff, compensated them well, and included them in process improvement. We had a wait list of people applying for nursing and APRN jobs. We were more productive than we'd ever been in the history of the agency. The staff was very happy and the complaints from staff and patients slowed to a trickle. I then proposed to leadership that my position be made official and was promoted to director, working alongside the physician medical director (who had different responsibilities). This is an example of recognizing the void in the system (high turnover, low employee satisfaction, unsustainable workload) and being a positive disruptor (nurse creating leadership roles in a space typically filled by physicians).

The ladder of engagement can help illustrate how every nurse can lean into leadership, broaden their influence, and capitalize on the fraternity of the nursing profession. This ladder of engagement approach still requires the nurse to understand what type of leader they are, recognize voids in systems, and fill the voids by being a positive disruptor. See also Table 1.1 and Table 5.1.

Level 1: Unaware—Unaware of the issues or have accepted the status (students, novices)

Level 2: Aware, unengaged—Aware of the issues; do not participate in addressing them

Level 3: Minimally engaged—Unlikely to engage online; may participate in online activities if convenient

Level 4: Moderately engaged—Passively engaged online; may participate in an in-person event if convenient

Level 5: Highly engaged—Seek out opportunities to engage online, likely to engage in person, will participate if the pathway is created, seek out and address issues

Level 6: Activist—Change agents directly engaged in advocacy, policy making, and creating dialogue. These are highly visible entrepreneurs, innovators, and leaders who create engagement opportunities for self and others and seek out and engage issues. For example, students and practicing nurses at levels 1 and 2 may be unaware of their ability to lead.

Table 5.1 Leadership and Level of Engagement

Level	Individual	Institutional	National and International
1, 2	Understand leadership type	x	x
3, 4	Understand leadership type	Assert change	x
5, 6	Understand leadership type	Assert change	Create mass direction

Every nursing school curriculum should include leadership training (not to be confused with management training). The goal of this training should be to introduce pathways to leadership at the individual, institutional, regional, and national levels. Nurses who are not in formal leadership positions should familiarize themselves with leadership styles, specifically the leadership styles of those within their institution, as well as any gaps within the structure. Once comfortable at levels 1 and 2, nurses should move to levels 3 and 4.

Nurses at levels 3 and 4 may be in lower (i.e., charge nurse) to executive level leadership (i.e., chief nursing officer). These nurses should consider and evaluate their leadership style and familiarize themselves with the leadership structure within their institution as well as any gaps within the structure. These nurses are positioned to assert themselves as change agents within their health system. As change agents, these nurses seek to create positive and sustainable culture shifts that empower subordinates and peers. These nurses should push the boundaries of their leadership roles by being positive disruptors. I have witnessed a great deal of unjustified angst when nurses reach the leadership table. This may be an acceptable barrier for the novice leader; however, in order for nurses to truly lead, we must be prepared to take bold and decisive action. When posed with the option to "do the right thing" it is better to ask for forgiveness than permission.

Nurses at levels 5 and 6 are at the national and international leadership levels and may be well established nurse scientists, leaders of professional organizations, and established change agents.

These nurses often understand leadership well and know what type of leader they are as well as how to assert change within institutions and systems. These nurses are influential within their sphere and in prime position to direct a nation on healthcare-related strategies. However, the general population does not seek information from these nurses. These nurses are rarely front and center during a national, international, or systemic health crisis, even though these nurses are in an optimal position to lead and direct healthcare and planning on a mass scale. These nurses are also in prime position to amplify their impact by forming coalitions with other nursing organizations, disrupting the status quo, and revolutionizing healthcare.

NURSING POWER

Similar to the literature on leadership, there is a plethora of information available about empowerment, specifically nurse empowerment. Despite all of this information being readily available, nurses consistently report feeling powerless (Adkins, n.d.). Traditional nursing professional culture does not promote individual or collective empowerment. Nurses are trained to advocate for patients. In general, nurses are not encouraged, trained, or empowered to advocate for themselves, their colleagues, the nursing profession, or the general public. If, by chance, a nurse is empowered enough to advocate beyond the bedside, rest assured they have arrived at this juncture through sheer determination.

Disempowerment Factors

Nurses consistently describe feeling as if they are unable to make significant changes in their professional lives. There are several reasons why nurses feel disempowered. Factors include but are not limited to a professional culture that does not promote empowerment, competing personal and professional interests, a constant need to mitigate risks, and culturally ingrained cynicism.

Professional Culture: Many aspects of professional nursing culture are the antithesis to empowerment. On a systemic level, the concerns of nurses are largely ignored. Nurses are constantly understaffed, underpaid, overworked, disrespected, and mistreated. Aside from collective bargaining agencies, there are only a few weak internal mechanisms that can check the power of the healthcare system in any meaningful way. From a cultural perspective, it is common practice to offer pizza or other small tokens of appreciation to worn out and demoralized nursing staff. It is common for disempowered nursing staff to reach the breaking point. Soon after, the rumors that the staff has contracted a case of "the quits" start to circulate. There are few things that more clearly convey the message that people don't have any power than management's providing a slice of terrible cold pizza to quell the rumblings of disgruntled staff. As silly as this sounds, it is a common practice that plays out over and over again in healthcare facilities throughout the United States. Finally, on an individual level, nursing culture is inundated with undermining and self-defeating practices that constantly inhibit progress (e.g., lateral violence and bullying). It is difficult to feel empowered in an environment where colleagues battle about everything, nothing at all, and all in between.

Competing Interests: A major barrier to nurses becoming empowered are competing interests of family life. Nurses, most of whom are women, are constantly fighting battles on two fronts: home life and work life. Nurses may know what the problems are in healthcare and likely have thought of solutions to the problems. However, when the decision to devote energy to taking professional action is juxtaposed against devoting energy to a family, naturally most people will choose family first.

Mitigating Risk: In addition to navigating competing interests, nurses must mitigate risk associated with taking any stance beyond the status quo. Nurses, particularly those who work in right-to-work states or do not have union protections, often find themselves in the precarious situation of deciding if speaking up is worth losing their job. This is why despite there being "regulations" outlining rules for nurse work environments, those rules are seldom followed, and almost no one ever reports when rules are broken. Many nurses are stuck between staying in a bad job and getting fired for trying to improve it. Lastly, job loss is on the extreme end of risk mitigation. Loss of career momentum is also a risk that many nurses are not willing to take.

Cynicism: Cynical attitudes are pervasive in nursing culture. This is not limited to any demographic or age group. I can't count how many times I've heard a seasoned nurse say, "It's been this way forever," followed by, "Nothing will change." The millennial generation tends to view careers differently than other generations; they are the least likely generation to stay with a single employer long term and the most likely generation to change jobs frequently (American Sentinel University, 2017). This is not necessarily a negative culture shift but rather a reflection of how a generation of people has shifted from focusing on work to focusing on self-interests. The result is a hopeless senior generation and a younger generation that isn't interested in wasting energy on fruitless efforts.

Pathways to Empowerment

As nurses, we must know and understand the rules of engagement before we can empower or be empowered. Empowerment in nursing starts with our own individual practices. This is where nurses are most comfortable. In order to truly revolutionize healthcare, nurses must extend this power beyond the bedside to our colleagues, our institutions, our local communities, and throughout the world.

Practice: Every nurse has the opportunity to be a leader in their individual practice. However, before we can be an exemplar of good nursing practice, we must know "the rules" of our practice—in other words, know the job and the role within the team as well as the expectations of colleagues and patients. Most important, every nurse should know and understand the scope of practice as decreed by their local board of nursing. I cannot emphasize this last point enough.

Many nurses have been reported to their board of nursing after an unintentional infraction. For example, I once worked at a practice where I was fairly well known and liked (presumably). In this practice I was formally recognized as a leader, an exemplar of professionalism and good clinical practice. A colleague at this same practice confided in me that they wanted to seek medical care for a condition but could not afford a visit with their primary care provider. The colleague asked me to treat them. I collected the necessary medical history and gave them a prescription. I had observed my physician and APRN colleagues treating other colleagues as a common practice. However, I had unknowingly broken the law. I had performed care without documenting the encounter, which is illegal in my state. I was thus reported to the board of nursing. The investigation led to remediation (learning laws and statutes pertinent to my practice), a probationary period, and a permanent mark on my license. The moral of this story is that I was an exemplary employee who was attempting to help a colleague. My intentions were good. However, my ignorance of the legal practice authority had real consequences. My own ignorance tarnished my role as a stellar employee, advocate, and clinician.

Through this experience I learned that, as nurses, we cannot win the game if we don't know the rules. Fortunately, I also learned more about the scope of my practice. Importantly, I learned that the board of nursing makes the rules for nursing practice in each state, and it is up to each individual nurse to be familiar with these rules. In this situation, it wasn't enough for me to be satisfied with being a good clinician or being helpful to my colleagues. Had I known and fully understood the rules of engagement, I would have had a greater chance of having a positive impact. In order to truly be powerful in a space, we must know the rules of the space we occupy.

Colleagues: Healthcare is hierarchical by design. There are administrators who manage staff and facilities; interns, residents, and attending physicians who give orders; charge nurses and unit managers; and a constant stream of novices and student learners. It takes years for the novice to truly understand all of the roles in a healthcare team and sometimes longer to understand who truly holds power. It is a curious thing to figure out who, of all the people milling around a healthcare facility, has power and who has influence. Power and influence are not synonymous in these settings. An administrator may seem powerful if they are listed as a "Director of XYZ Department"; however, it may be the nurse with 25 years of experience who has the greatest influence over the environment and the team.

I once worked as a staff nurse with a charge nurse we called "Scary Mary." She was terrifying. Scary Mary presented as a traditional middle-aged veteran nurse and she ran a very tight ship. I was a young male nurse with a patchy beard and dreadlocks that hung midway down my back. To say we came from different worlds would be an understatement. Every day that I worked on Scary Mary's unit I thought to myself, "I don't think I can work with this lady."

I watched the staff scurry and jump to attention when she gave orders. I noticed that the physicians gave her their full attention when she spoke. The patients seemed to know that her word was the last word. Nevertheless, I fell in line like everyone else on her unit. Over time, I got to know Scary Mary, and I learned that she was not scary at all. Her work was impeccable. She was respected and her influence was powerful. To some people, she was intimidating. Staff who couldn't "hack it" on Scary Mary's floor were magically assigned to different units. Everyone else fell in line. I enjoyed the work but was at my wit's end with Scary Mary's military precision.

One day I asked Scary Mary to give me an explanation for an order she gave me. She answered factually, and it wasn't scary at all. I decided to ask her to teach me more of what she knew, and to my surprise she did so happily. She taught me her rules, methods, and tricks. Eventually, I stopped asking but she kept giving me her little pearls. When it was time for a charge nurse to be trained for a different unit, my name came up. I excitedly told Scary Mary about my promotion, to which she replied, "Yes, I know. Who do you think told them to put you there?"

When I started working at Scary Mary's hospital, I completed new employee orientation. I learned who all of the bosses were. I learned about all of the "important" people in the hospital, but no one told me about Scary Mary. It would take me 2 years to understand all of the players in the hospital, such as who had power and who had influence. I learned that the people who have power and influence in healthcare settings are not always who we expect. The moral of this story is not to get chummy with people who can help your career (though that doesn't hurt). Instead, the moral of the story is that it is important for nurses to empower each other. It is equally important for every nurse to know and understand the visible and invisible leadership structures in which they work, who holds power, who holds influence, and who holds both.

Institutions: In many ways, healthcare professionals work and operate on a need-to-know basis within their healthcare institutions. Regardless of the size of the healthcare facility or institution, we are expected to show up, do our work, and avoid meddling in anything that isn't our responsibility. We've all heard a colleague say, "That's not my job." Whether we cringed when we heard the words or agreed with the sentiment, we understood that our colleague believed in staying in their lane.

Healthcare is moving toward more integrative and interdisciplinary care team models. Yet our view of the healthcare institution is often limited to our most proximal colleagues, staff, and workflows. This way of being in the workplace is problematic for many reasons. First, our view is limited. Think of the viewpoint of the eagle and a beaver living in the same habitat. When an eagle soars high above a field, they can see miles into the distance in multiple directions. They can see storms approaching as well as other animals moving on land and in the air. They can see the movements of small animals on the ground. They can see features of the landscape like hills, valleys, waterways, and fields. The eagle knows all of the borders of the terrain and can oversee the entire ecosystem.

The beaver, in contrast, can see the stream of water, the dam they built, and the pond they cultivated. They can see their home made of logs and all of the other animals that inhabit their small pond. Indeed, the beaver knows nearly everything about the pond.

The beaver view, being close to the ground and deep within the habitat, helps the beaver find and secure its needs. Similarly, the eagle view, being high above the habitat, helps it find and secure its needs. However, the eagle knows little about the beaver pond, and the beaver has never seen the mountains in the distance. The viewpoints of the eagle and the beaver are useful, but neither fully understands or can even conceptualize the other's viewpoint.

Nurses, like other healthcare professionals, often work like beavers. In this scenario, their view of the institution (or the ecosystem) is often limited to their daily workflows at worst or workflows within the institution at best. When a beaver makes a dam, they are not concerned with subsequently flooding an adjacent field or displacing other animals. They are just doing their work. As nurses, we are often "too busy" to be concerned with the larger ecosystem and don't actually see beyond our daily work.

Meanwhile, the eagle knows that the beaver built the dam, which created the pond that supplies fish for its consumption. However, the eagle cannot see the granular details of the beaver dam. The eagle is unaware of how much effort the beaver used to build its home or what the beaver does on a day-to-day basis. Healthcare institutional leaders are like eagles. They can see far and wide but can rarely connect with or appreciate what's happening on the ground. This disconnect between leadership and frontline employees happens in many industries and is not unique to nursing. The point of this analogy is that the nurses within a healthcare institution cannot be empowered unless the people with the eagle view and the people with the beaver view are the same people. To empower the profession of nursing, more bedside nurses need to assume leadership roles, and they must never forget the view from the bedside.

National and International: There are countless nongovernmental organizations working to relieve illness and improve health around the United States and around the world. Considering how many nurses make up the healthcare workforce, very few healthcare organizations are nurse led or offer the nursing approach to solve complex health problems. There are few nurses leading national or global health efforts. The United Nations has almost no nurse-led global initiatives. There are no nurse positions a person can be appointed to at the federal level in the United States. Occasionally, a nurse is elected to Congress. However, Congress does not have a committee dedicated to health. There are no nurses on the U.S. Senate's health education, labor, and pensions committees. Despite the contributions of nurses to the health and well-being of nearly all of the humans on the planet, it is quite uncommon to see nurses empowered, visible in the public eye, and at the leadership table with heads of state.

The World Health Organization (WHO) declared 2020 the year of the nurse. Yet there are few nurse-led initiatives anywhere in the world. The national and international power of nurses is as invisible as the leadership positions we've never been allowed to have. If we want to empower nurses through our institutions, communities, nations, and the world, we must ensure they see themselves reflected as leaders at every level of leadership.

CONCLUSION

The levels of engagement model is a good way to conceptualize how every nurse is a leader and has potential for leadership beyond the bedside. The levels in this instance include examining and learning preferred leadership style, asserting change at the institutional level, and asserting change at the national and international levels. Regardless of where a nurse is on the ladder of engagement, they can move to the next level and should encourage other nurses to do so as well.

There are several factors that disempower nurses, including negative aspects of nursing culture, competing interests, need to mitigate risk, and cynicism. Every nurse should engage and dismantle negative nursing culture, promote a culture that diminishes bullying, reject cynicism, and generally build a more supportive collegial culture within the nursing profession.

Regardless of how busy their home life is, every nurse can engage in small meaningful ways that help elevate the nursing profession. A nurse who is being kind and supportive to their colleague and the nurse who is elected to Congress are both empowering and revolutionizing the profession. Every positive action beyond the bedside is important.

Similarly, it is essential that nurses know the limits of their professional boundaries. We cannot be empowered or empower others if we do not know the rules and laws that govern our practice. Every nurse must know where they've been, where they are, and where they're going professionally. Empowerment cannot happen without direction.

In order to truly be powerful in a space, we must know the rules of the space we occupy. A direct path to empowering nurses in practice includes being well versed in and fully understanding the laws that govern practice as dictated by the board of nursing. Every nurse should not only know the laws that govern their practice but should be able to help others understand these rules as well.

It is important for nurses to empower each other as well as to be well acquainted with the visible and invisible leadership structures in their institutions. To have influence we must understand who holds power, who holds influence, and who holds both.

Nurses who have moved from the bedside to leadership have an excellent vantage point from which to empower other nurses. More bedside nurses need to assume executive-level leadership roles from which they can lift the system, their colleagues, and the profession at large. Lastly, if we truly want to empower nurses we must ensure that nursing leaders are highly visible at the institutional, community, state, federal, and global leadership levels.

DISCUSSION AND REFLECTION POINTS

1. What is your level of engagement as a leader?
2. What is your preferred leadership style?

3. Are there any disempowering or competing interests that prevent you from being a more influential leader?
4. What is your typical reaction to cynicism in the workplace?
5. Review your local board of nursing website.
   a. Did you find anything surprising?
6. Who are the official leaders in your institution?
   a. Who are the unofficial leaders in your institution?
7. Name a nurse in leadership.
   a. Institution level
   b. Regional level
   c. State level
   d. Federal level
   e. National level
   f. Global level

REFERENCES

Adkins, A. (n.d.). *Millennials: The job-hopping generation.* https://www.gallup.com/workplace/231587/millennials-job-hopping-generation.aspx

American Sentinel University. (2017). Secrets of effective nurse leaders: EMPOWERMENT. *The Sentinel Watch.* https://www.americansentinel.edu/blog/2017/05/09/secrets-of-effective-nurse-leaders-empowerment/

6

Self-Advocacy Beyond the Bedside

INTRODUCTION

Throughout this chapter I discuss and use the term "nurse self-advocacy." The term "self-advocacy" is self-explanatory. However, when I mention self-advocacy, I am referring to self-advocacy beyond the bedside specifically. This is an important distinction, as nurses are introduced to advocacy very early in their training. This training is patient-centric, with nearly every aspect of advocacy revolving around the patient, ensuring their needs are met and they are safe. Nurses simply are not taught to advocate for themselves. I would venture so far as to say that the culture of nursing and healthcare suggest that nurses should not only advocate for their patients but they should sacrifice their own well-being to ensure their patients are cared for. Surely, this selfless culture lends to the nobility nurses have earned in the public eye. For nearly two decades, nursing has been ranked as the most trusted profession. This is because the public knows a nurse will hold their bladder for hours just to take care of their patients, they may not eat all day while working, or they may get spattered with someone's bodily fluids and continue to care for the person. This list could go on and on. The point is that self-advocacy is not reflected within healthcare or within nursing specifically, and neither the healthcare industry nor the public expects nurses to self-advocate in any significant way. This chapter is about shifting that narrative within nursing, within healthcare, and within broader society.

I was not introduced to nurse self-advocacy until late in my career; even then, it was purely accidental. In September of 2015, I was midway through completing my second advanced degree (PhD) and was comfortably working as an APN in an outpatient clinic. I was also relatively far removed from the bedside at this point in my career. During that time I was invited to join a Facebook group called Show Me Your Stethoscope, which was started in response to media personalities insulting a nurse and quickly grew to hundreds of thousands of nurses from all around the United States (in some cases, the world), from different cultural backgrounds, with different political affiliations, with different education, and with different religious and philosophical backgrounds. There were two things that bound all of these nurses together: (a) nursing and (b) a call to do more as a profession. As I watched the comments stream into the group, these themes were consistent and persistent. Nurses told stories of feeling undervalued, underpaid, abused, overworked, mistreated, and burned out. The call to action was palpable, but the methodology to mobilize online communities was absent. This is what drew me back to nursing and convinced me to reinvest in doing whatever I could to help the bedside nurse. Over the years, I watched individual bedside nurses within this online community organize themselves and mobilize to advocate for themselves. These bedside nurses really helped me understand what nurse self-advocacy was, what it wasn't, and why so many nurses like me left the bedside.

Ineffective Self-Advocacy Causes Burnout

Nurses leave the bedside for many reasons, but a common one is burnout. Compassion fatigue, which is a diminished ability to empathize or feel compassion, which can be a negative effect of providing care, also affects nurses. However, while the symptoms of compassion fatigue and burnout may appear similar, their etiology is in fact different. Compassion fatigue is related to secondary traumatic stress related to care giving. There are nursing campaigns aimed at reducing compassion fatigue, by encouraging nurses to actively engage in self-care. Nurses should engage in self-care behaviors. However, nurses are leaving the bedside as a result of burnout, not compassion fatigue. Burnout is related to unrealistic workloads, lack of control, lack of support, and, most important, powerlessness. Burnout can be a direct result of powerlessness and feeling as if there are no options to change a situation for the better. The inability to effectively self-advocate leads to burnout, which leads to nurses leaving the bedside in droves.

I was one of the frustrated nurses who left the bedside. I remember so many scary situations, far too many close calls, and feeling like it was impossible to do my job the way I was trained to do it. Most of all, I felt as if there was nothing I could do to change any of the way the healthcare system worked. Therefore, I did what any reasonable nurse would do: I changed specialties. I even changed practice settings and earned advanced degrees. Still, as far as being powerless was concerned, nothing really changed.

These same issues followed me irrespective of where I worked—being unsupported, feeling underappreciated for my work, suffering from high burnout, and facing dangerous clinical situations. I felt I couldn't help people the way I was told I would be able to when I was in school.

I didn't want to change professions entirely. Choosing nursing for my profession saved my life in so many ways, gave me purpose, and helped me become a responsible contributing member of society. Therefore, despite the problems in our profession, I owe much of my good fortune to nursing. I wasn't ready to walk away, but I couldn't tolerate the powerless feeling that haunted me.

Example: Self-Advocacy and Nurse Staffing

There are three topics that every nurse, irrespective of specialty, education, or practice setting, will agree on: unsafe staffing, unsafe workloads, and burnout. Of the many issues nurses can and should advocate for, these are the topics that most bedside nurses agree are problematic for individual nurses, the nursing profession, and healthcare at large. These topics also give us near perfect examples of the untapped power nurses have within the healthcare industry.

There is overwhelming evidence that unsafe staffing negatively impacts patient outcomes, nursing care, and nursing staff (Department for Professional Employees, 2019). This is a well-known, well-documented problem in healthcare. Moreover, regardless of which side of healthcare we fall on (consumer or practitioner) and regardless of our level of nursing practice, unsafe staffing will affect us all at some point. This is our reality as healthcare providers and consumers.

Maintaining safe staffing ratios is not a new concept. Many industries, such as airlines and day-care providers, regulate the number of staff required to safely take care of consumers (patients). These practices have been incredibly elusive for the nursing profession. However, this is not to say that there haven't been efforts to address the problem of nurse staffing. There are literally hundreds of state, national, and international nursing organizations. Every nursing organization is aware of the problems associated with nurse staffing. Any healthcare institution in the United States that employs nurses is intimate aware of the problems associated with nurse staffing. Most important, every nurse (>3 million RNs, >800,000 LPNs, >1.5 million certified nursing assistants [CNAs]) is aware of the problems associated with nurse staffing. Still, aside from a few states that have managed to pass state nurse staffing laws and those facilities with a nursing union, nearly the entire workforce of nurses in the United States is being crushed by this problem.

If safe staffing legislation is an overarching problem affecting many aspects of healthcare and all aspects of nursing, then we have to ask the question, "Why can't nurses fix staffing problems?" I'll tell you why. It has nothing to do with the methods of fixing the staffing problem (unions, legislation, etc.). It is our inability to unite around this issue that prevents us from fixing the problem. This disunity is ingrained and deeply entrenched in our professional culture. Nurses do want to fix the obvious problems in healthcare and in nursing. Yet we can't see our dysfunction despite the repeated gut punches it gives us every time we try to fight against it.

This disunity is slow growing and ever present. This malignant separatism within our professional culture defeats us at every turn. It is planted within us early in our career as students, then is reared and fed as we become new nurses, matures over time as we gain experience, and finally is harvested to be replanted through the training of nurse leaders. You see, in nursing culture, there is always an "us" versus "them," waiting to rear its ugly head and prevent progress. These are the age old divisive arguments—RN versus LPN, ADN versus BSN, NP versus DNP, DNP versus PhD, staff versus management, new nurses versus experienced nurses, specialty versus subspecialty, professional organization versus subspecialty organization, union versus nonunion, and so on. These outdated ideas are counterproductive fossils, yet we cradle and feed them like precious infants. We grow them, and they turn into the monsters that eat us.

When it comes to unifying and self-advocacy, we are both the problem and the solution to the problem. Our profession is plagued with larger-than-life egos and self-righteousness. We have hundreds of professional organizations and unions, all self-serving and grasping, clawing, and contending with each other. Each has their own version of exclusivity, vying for a validity and a reason to be needed. Each claims to be the "voice" for nurses; however, none put their money where their mouth is and actually bring ALL nurses together. To be fair, they don't all share the same mission and goals; however, they have proven to be wholly ineffective at uniting the profession.

The result of the fractured nursing profession is that the individual voices of nurses are not amplified. Individual nurses who feel muted eventually burn out and leave the bedside. This problematic culture ultimately has consequences for the entire healthcare system.

Example: Consequences of Nursing Cultural Dysfunction

There are many examples throughout recent history of nurses being defeated by the healthcare industry. A perfect example of how nursing culture has prevented nurses from actualizing their individual, professional, industry, and societal power is best illustrated by the way Massachusetts nurses were defeated in 2018.

The Massachusetts Nurses Association (MNA) attempted, for many years, to help ensure that hospitals in Massachusetts were staffed safely. In 2014, the MNA was able to get a landmark law passed for the state limiting the number of patients a nurse can be assigned in the ICU. This meant it was against Massachusetts state law for a hospital to assign more than two patients to one ICU nurse. This ensured nurses would not get burned out by overwhelming workloads and leave the bedside; more important, patients would receive excellent care.

The MNA tried working with state legislators to pass other laws mandating limits on the number of patients assigned to a nurse in other settings. However, powerful lobbyists associated with Massachusetts hospitals also worked with state legislators and were able to prevent these drafts from ever making it out of the legislative committee to the floor for a vote. The MNA then attempted to add their safe patient limits campaign on the November 2018 ballot as a question for the Massachusetts voters to answer.

The safe patient limits ballot question in Massachusetts initiated by nurses did not pass. The question was simple. It was not worded poorly or confusing. The question was, "Should nurses have a limit on the number of patients they can be assigned in a hospital?"

If presented without any additional influential context, the public would have voted to support this question being adopted into law. No reasonable person would want a nurse to have too many patients to care for. However, the powerful hospital association lobbyist ran a very effective negative ad campaign that literally terrified the public, and some nurses, with threats of hospitals closing due to inability to staff properly (Massachusetts is one of the few states without a nursing shortage, with 3,000 graduating annually), long ED wait times, layoffs, and so on. By the time the public got to the voting booth, they were terrified.

Hospital Associations

You might be wondering why hospital associations would be against nurses. As we discussed in Chapter 4, medical providers, like physicians, are revenue generators for a hospital. They bill for services and the hospital makes money. Nurses, on the other hand, are considered an expense, a line item like a mop or a light bulb. Hospitals view nurses as an expense to be managed. So, from a business perspective, hospitals want to get as much work out of each nurse as possible. If there are laws with limits to the number of patients a hospital can assign a nurse, that law would cut into their net profits. The way the hospital views this is, "Why pay one nurse to care for five patients when we can pay one nurse to take care of 10 patients?"

The hospital associations' "public" argument was that the law would be costly and wouldn't improve outcomes. Additionally, there were some legitimate arguments against mandated nurse-to-patient ratios. For instance, most nurses believed that acuity should be considered when staffing a unit (the Massachusetts law allowed hospital unit administrators to adjust for acuity). Regardless, the hospital association lobbyists' work was to ensure that hospitals and healthcare systems were able to push the limits of nurse staffing and that no law was put in place to prevent this practice.

The Massachusetts hospital associations and lobbyists spent $25 million on scare tactics and negative ads to beat the nurses of Massachusetts, and it worked. After the MNA was defeated, I had so many questions. What happened to the nurses? How did money beat the largest workforce within the healthcare industry? How did money beat the people?

I read as much as I could about the ballot question before and after the vote. I talked to nurses in Massachusetts and around the United States. I really wanted to understand how this happened.

Lobbyist Wars

Massachusetts has world renowned healthcare. The negative ad campaign by the hospital associations was so effective that it convinced the public that "the government" would wreck the very good healthcare system in Massachusetts. Some people were so confused that they thought the ballot question was a terrible "government mandate," because they knew some nurses who were against it. The negative ads were so convincing that some people, including nurses, literally didn't know that the bill was written by nurses.

Some nurses argued the ballot question wasn't written perfectly. I disagree with this as a reason not to support nurses. Whatever legislators didn't like about the bill could have been amended. Another argument was that the law was too drastic, and hospitals would close due to their inability to comply. One of the scare tactics used by the hospital association was to promote an idea that hospitals had to be compliant with the new law within 30 days or be fined $25,000 per infraction. This was found to be wholly untrue as drafted law literally allowed legislators years to implement the law and hospitals had years of grace periods allowing them to staff appropriately.

The nurses who didn't like the law proposed in the ballot question typically had no real solutions to the problems of unsafe staffing and nurse burnout. Many nurses believed the negative hype suggested from the hospital

143

association and voted against their own interests. Their friends, families, and neighbors followed suit.

In the end, I drew a simple conclusion as to what happened and how the nurses were defeated. Simply put, nurses, the most trusted profession in the world, were not unified behind the effort. What happened instead was the typical union versus nonunion debate, followed by the management versus bedside debate, and then the big hospitals versus small hospitals debate; finally, the progressives and conservatives dug their heels in at the end. This drama played out at the organizational level as well, with the American Nurses Association (ANA) coming out against the ballot question, which was sponsored by a nursing union, the MNA.

You might be wondering: Why would two nursing organizations oppose each other publicly, especially when both organizations proclaim to speak for and advocate for nurses? The MNA was previously affiliated with the ANA but split from the national organization in 2001. According to the MNA, the reason for the split from the ANA included "concerns about the ANA . . . being too moderate and slow to respond to a growing crisis in nursing, including the impact of managed care, health care corporatization, short staffing, mandatory overtime and other issues causing turmoil for nurses at the bedside" (MNA, 2001, para. 3).

This is a recent example of nursing organizations undermining, undercutting, publicly disagreeing, and ultimately helping nurses to their defeat. However, this is not a new phenomenon. This is a systemic, cultural illness within nursing, an old, predictable, and quite frankly bizarre story of how we nurses consistently undermine our own interests.

At the end of this saga, Massachusetts nurses, the largest and most trusted workforce in the great healthcare systems of Massachusetts, did not unite behind this ballot question. Using the divide and conquer strategy and millions of dollars in negative ads, the hospital association lobbyists were able to snuff out the Massachusetts nurses.

The Massachusetts nurses may have had a spark of fire left after fighting with the lobbyists, but whatever fire was left was extinguished by the public squabbling by the two prominent professional organizations who claim to represent nurses in the state. On voting day, nurses were not marching to the polls toward a victory. Many nurses supported the ballot question, but most of the public, and some nurses, were still scurrying, confused, disoriented, and unsure if the ballot question was good or a terrible mistake.

There are 150,000 nurses in Massachusetts. If each nurse agreed with the ballot question and convinced 20 friends and family to vote yes for the ballot question, that would have been 3 million yes votes (Massachusetts only has 6.8 million residents). This is an example of how shortsightedness prevented nurses from making a real stand in one of the greatest healthcare systems in the world.

The shortsightedness was not just limited to nurses in Massachusetts. Millions of nurses around the United States could have supported the nurses in Massachusetts. Unfortunately, most nurses around the United States did not know what was happening with the Massachusetts ballot question, nor did they understand the significance of the question. Our professional organizations around the country did very little to support these nurses in Massachusetts.

Nurses are notoriously easy to beat when it comes to self-advocacy beyond the bedside because of how fractioned the profession is. The culture of professional nursing is such that most nurses tend to sit in silos and complain. I call this complacent complaining. Few nurses advocate for other nurses practicing outside of their specialty area (e.g., hospital nurses don't advocate for nursing home nurses) or practicing at a different level (primary care NPs generally don't advocate for ED nurses) and almost never support nurses practicing in another state. This shortsightedness and self-sabotage is our problem in nursing. We are our greatest asset and our own worst enemy.

The effect of this cultural dysfunction within nursing is that it breeds individual dysfunction, which in turn leads to professional dysfunction and ultimately dysfunction within the healthcare system. When an individual cannot effectively self-advocate, the profession cannot effectively self-advocate, and if nurses do not self-advocate, healthcare will continue to worsen for everyone.

In conclusion, the nursing profession has a weak culture of self-advocacy and a nonexistent culture of self-advocacy beyond the bedside. Professional nursing organizations fracture slivers of the nursing community and do a great disservice to the profession by potentiating division. Finally, there can be no collective nursing influence within the profession, healthcare, or the world at large without a significant cultural shift toward a unified profession.

Moving Self-Advocacy Forward

Traditionally, nurses have advocated for themselves through brick-and-mortar institutions. These include unions, trade associations, and professional organizations. These institutions typically have traditional corporate or shared governance leadership models, physical locations, and some criteria for membership.

Professional Organizations

There are hundreds of professional organizations in the United States. Some well-known organizations include the ANA and the National League of Nurses. These organizations are managed by nurses and boards of directors, all of whom are elected by their members. Criteria for membership is based on paying dues, licensure, and education. Typically, these organizations have a headquarters and regional or state branches, which may also require dues. Generally, membership rates for these types of nursing organizations are in a steady decline. However, very large professional organizations like the ANA do not require a substantial member base (ANA membership represents less than 5% of U.S. nurses) to remain financially viable. This is because much of the ANA's over $45 million annual budget is comprised of diverse revenue streams such as credentialing and accrediting for both individuals and institutions. These kinds of organizations are relatively well connected to lawmakers at the state and national levels. They tend to dedicate some revenues toward lobbying and work directly with other lobbying institutions like the American Hospital Association, an organization that represents the interests of over 5,000 hospitals in the United States.

The problem with professional organizations is that they create an exclusive community while claiming to represent the entire population of nurses. Additionally, the leadership in these organizations tends to be viewed as an ivory tower institution that looks down on the common nurse. Most nurses do not feel represented by the large nursing organizations. If you ask any LPN working a night shift in a long-term care facility with an assignment of 40 patients if any of the large professional nursing organizations represent their interests, I assure you they will report that these organizations do not represent their interests.

Specialty Nursing Organizations

Specialty nursing organizations are structured and function similarly to the professional organizations described earlier. However, these organizations tend to represent a niche nursing community that may emphasize ethnicity (National Black Nurses Association, National Association of Hispanic Nurses), specialty practice (Emergency Nurses Association, National Association of School Nurses, The American Association of Nurse Practitioners), licensure (National Association of Licensed Practical Nurses, National Association of Healthcare Assistants), or education (Eastern Nursing Research Society, The Association of Community Health Nursing Educators). Specialty nursing organizations, though structured similarly to larger, less specific organizations, by nature tend to be smaller (fewer members, smaller budgets) and focused on affecting change in their small niche area. These organizations tend to be less effective and generally not focused on advocating for the general population of nurses.

The problem with specialty nursing organizations is that they are, by default, exclusive. These organizations may be helpful in some respects by catering to a small subset of the general nursing population; however, they do a great disservice by fractioning what could be a large and powerful collective. Ultimately, this weakens advocacy efforts as these organizations detract by pulling nurses' efforts away from the general nursing population.

Labor Unions

Labor unions, commonly known as unions, are associations comprised of workers who form a collective bargaining unit to represent their interests to an employer. Leadership structures within nursing unions tend to be comprised of elected and appointed representatives. Some nursing unions are large, powerful, and independent, such as the California Nurses Association. Other large and powerful unions, such as the American Federation of Teachers and the American Federation of

Labor and Congress of Industrial Organization (AFL-CIO), have a nursing or healthcare division. Criteria for nurse union membership are typically related to the state laws and hospital policy. Some hospitals require that nurses become union members and pay union dues.

The history of labor unions in the world and in the United States is complicated. However, the current view of nursing unions in the United States can best be understood by understanding the history and dynamics between employers and unions—the pros versus cons of labor unions and right-to-work versus not right-to-work states. The National Labor Relations Act of 1935 is a labor law allowing private sector employees to organize into trade unions and engage in collective bargaining. Collective bargaining is the process of negotiating between employers and employees and may include coming to agreements on topics such as wages, working hours, benefits, and safety. Unions have been associated with improving conditions, safety, and pay for workers as well as increasing the cost of doing business.

Nursing unions are controversial in that hospitals prefer not to be unionized. Generally, the hospitals argue, and rightly so to some degree, that unions drive up the cost of employing nurses. This happens as a direct result of nursing unions using collective bargaining to gain better wages and benefits. Without collective bargaining, the hospital is able to offer the lowest pay and the least costly benefit packages to their staff. Some hospital systems spend exorbitant amounts of money to prevent unionization and defeat collective bargaining negotiations by nurses. The nurse unions will argue that through collective bargaining they are able to protect workers from being abused by the employer, negotiate better work environments, reduce staff turnover, and improve outcomes.

States that have right-to-work laws do not require union membership as a condition of employment and tend to have a weaker union presence and less cultural support for labor unions. Additionally, these states tend to be "at will" states, meaning the employer can terminate the employee so long as the reason for termination is not illegal. Generally, right-to-work states are in the south, southwest, and Midwestern parts of the United States and tend to be "red" or politically and culturally conservative states. These states include Alabama, Arkansas, Florida, Georgia, Idaho, Indiana, Iowa, Kansas, Kentucky, Louisiana, Michigan, Mississippi, Nebraska, Nevada, North Carolina, North Dakota, Oklahoma, South Carolina, South Dakota, Tennessee, Texas, Utah, Virginia, West Virginia, Wisconsin, and Wyoming.

States that do not have right-to-work laws allow union membership as a condition of employment and tend to have a stronger union presence and more cultural support for labor unions. These states tend to be located in the northeastern part of the United States, in the Midwest, and on the West Coast. Additionally, these states tend to be a combination of "red" and "blue" states, or politically and culturally conservative and/or progressive states. These states include California, Colorado, Connecticut, Illinois, Maine, Maryland, Massachusetts, Minnesota, Missouri, New Hampshire, New Jersey, New Mexico, New York, Ohio, Oregon, Pennsylvania, Rhode Island, Vermont, and Washington State.

The problem with nursing unions is they are not a one-size-fits-all solution. In some states with a progressive enough climate and culture, labor unions may be helpful. However, in states with right-to-work laws and more conservative culture and politics, labor unions are dirty words and likened to political suicide. While some idealists will reject the idea that unions are not the answer to the problems with nurse advocacy, there is ample proof that some parts of the United States will not accept collective bargaining as a solution to any kind of problem.

Additionally, there are formal opportunities within healthcare institutions for nurses to be involved in self-advocacy. Most larger hospitals have committees and subcommittees that work on special projects and solve local problems. These are opportunities for nurses to self-advocate on a small but likely palpable scale. Additionally, these opportunities allow nurses to showcase their value beyond the bedside, which can be beneficial to the nurse as well as to the institution.

The Online Versus Offline Myth

There are several misconceptions about self-advocacy beyond the bedside that prevent nurses from mobilizing. For instance, nurses may assume that a nursing agency is required or that people must meet in a physical space in order to be effective change agents. This is far from true. The age of information and the advent of social media have revolutionized everything we thought we knew about mobilizing people.

I was invited to the first Facebook leadership summit in Chicago in 2017. In his keynote address, Mark Zuckerberg described how the social media mega company interpreted market research that suggested brick-and-mortar communities (libraries, unions, professional organizations, etc.) were in steady decline, whereas social media communities were exploding at unprecedented rates. There are several reasons for this. First, free social media platforms allow people with vague affiliations or niche interests to come together. These connections are made easily despite geography, time zones, nationality, and cultural differences. Second, these communities and connections are free and easy to find. Third, advances in technology are such that nearly every person in the

United States walks around with a pocket computer (cell phone) that allows them to connect with anyone on earth at any time, as long as that person has access to a computer and the internet. There are many other reasons why online connections and communities have grown so rapidly. Considering these three reasons, it is easy to understand the appeal of using social media and the internet to form and find community.

Another misconception is that people spend time and do things either online or offline. This is far from true. Technology has become a seamless part of our everyday lives. Let's take a trip to the movies as an example. This may start with seeing an advertisement for a movie on a social media platform, then sending a text to a friend to see if they're interested in going to watch a movie, meeting in person to watch the movie with a friend, taking a selfie with the friend after the movie and posting it to an online platform, and then discussing the movie with friends online. In this example, it's easy to visualize how a person may engage in all these activities without "thinking" about whether they are doing something online or offline. Similarly, the world of advocacy has evolved to include online and offline activities.

Online Communities

Online nursing communities and advocacy have the potential to offer the same benefits and structure as brick-and-mortar organizations. The benefit of this type of organizational structure is the absence of physical barriers, time constraints, or geographical barriers. Social media companies continue to have limitations with their platforms, including problems with users monetizing on their platforms and users having limited control of the algorithms. However, the nature of these technology companies is that they must continue to evolve or be replaced by a competitor. This technology will only evolve and get better, and with it will come great opportunities for connectivity, community, and, of course, advocacy.

There are many examples of people using social media for advocacy. For example, every year professional nursing organizations bring hundreds of nurses to Washington, DC, to advocate for legislation that may be beneficial to nurses or patients. Bedside nurses from the online community Show Me Your Stethoscope teamed up with other nurses around the United States and, without any significant leadership experience or technology expertise, started using social media to organize an event called NursesTakeDC in 2016. These individuals have since mobilized thousands of nurses to fly themselves to Washington, DC, to advocate for federal safe staffing legislation, which, to date, has not been introduced. However, what is significant is that while powerful nursing organizations were able to arrange funding to transport nurses to Washington, DC, ordinary bedside nurses were able to empower and mobilize each other to do the same via a free social media platform. These nurses would go on to help other nurse-led causes, such as purchasing a tranquility room for trauma nurses who worked with the 2017 mass shooting in Las Vegas, sending nurses to West Africa to provide care to remote villages, sending aid to victims of Hurricane Harvey, and adopting hundreds of nurse families for Christmas (purchasing gifts for the family).

Outside of the healthcare industry, there are many examples of people using social media to create change. There are amazing communities that provide a range of supportive services not otherwise provided by industry, from discussing transformative dialogue about race through Be the Bridge (https://bethebridge.com), an online community by best-selling author Latasha Morrison, to communities like We All Believe In You (www.weallbelieveinyou. com/our-story) that help others get over their feelings of isolation associated with mental illness (by Blake Loates). These communities allow ordinary people to impact others in extraordinarily positive ways. One of my favorite social media advocacy communities is Female IN (FIN) (www.facebook.com/femaleing). This online community was founded by Lola Omolola and is primarily comprised of women in Africa. This community of over 1.7 million women is focused on supporting and nurturing women in communities where this kind of support is minimal or absent and has events in over 80 cities worldwide. I appreciate this social media community for the scale, organization, and ability to really mobilize people, but mostly I appreciate how a community of people decided to be their own salvation and help each other.

A Pathway to Better Self-Advocacy

Nurses can unite, advocate for themselves beyond the bedside, be effective, and become a powerful force within healthcare. However, we must first create the conditions for success. Three conditions are essential for nurses to effectively self-advocate beyond the bedside.

Condition 1: Unified Nursing Profession

The first and most important condition is that nurses are unified as a profession. This means removing any negative existing cultural barriers to unification. True nurse professional unification would mean nurses support each other irrespective of education, specialty, geographic location, political affiliation, religion, gender, or sexual orientation. This culture is possible to create. People who serve in the armed forces or in law enforcement work in service of and in fraternity with individuals who support each other. When this condition is met, the nurse with a PhD will actively support the LPN working in long-term care, the school nurse will support the ED nurse, and the ICU nurse will support the home health nurse. This kind of community will empower and lift the nursing profession to new heights.

Condition 2: Remove the Powerless Culture and Professional Dysfunction

The second condition is more of a cultural shift rooted in collectivism. The professional dysfunctions discussed in Chapter 3 must be removed from all aspects of nursing culture. Additionally, nurses are in a prime position to remove the old narrative of powerlessness. The truth is, while many nurses feel powerless, nurses are not actually powerless. This new narrative is something that must be spoken into truth and acted upon. The solution to the feelings of powerlessness is within each and every nurse. Nurses empowering and relying on self and each other is the answer to professional powerlessness. The path to power requires each nurse to lean into their power, retell their narrative as empowered and impactful, and take some control over their own individual and collective destiny. When enough nurses assert themselves as empowered self-advocates, the powerlessness narrative will fade into an old professional nursing chapter.

Condition 3: Scientific Nursing Consensus

The third condition is requiring a nursing professional and scientific consensus on past, present, and evolving problems in healthcare and society. Nurses in the United States are an incredibly diverse community. Additionally, nursing as a practice and science is incredibly diverse regarding the depth and breadth of topics the profession covers. When a controversial healthcare or social topic is brewing, nurses should have a readily available body of evidence demonstrating the nurse view and professional consensus. This consensus should be the guide for nurses as they navigate personal, professional, and civic responsibilities related to controversial topics. Without this published and readily available consensus, nurses may use information from other disciplines and possibly support a variety of initiatives, solutions, and paths to fixing problems.

CONCLUSION

Not every nurse needs to be a scientist, nor does every nurse need to be able to interpret high level science. However, every nurse should have access to the consensus and nursing position on modern issues. Nurse scientists, academic institutions, and professional organizations must use their influence and resources to consolidate and make the nursing consensus available to the general population. This available and digestible scientific nursing consensus is necessary if we are to empower all nurses in the United States. These conditions combined with the ladder of engagement can be a useful model to help move every nurse toward self-advocacy. As discussed in Chapter 1, less engaged nurses are on the lower rungs of the ladder; nurses become more engaged as they ascend the ladder, ultimately becoming activists at the top rung. Every nurse should engage in self-advocacy or professional advocacy beyond the bedside. The ladder of engagement can help every nurse in the United States move up a rung, thus becoming more engaged and ultimately transforming nursing and healthcare.

Level 1: Unaware—Unaware of the issues or have accepted the status (students, novices)

Level 2: Aware, unengaged—Aware of the issues; do not participate in addressing them

Level 3: Minimally engaged—May participate in online activities if convenient

Level 4: Moderately engaged—Passive online engagement; participate in person if convenient

Level 5: Highly engaged—Seek out opportunities to engage online; likely to engage in person

Level 6: Activist—Change agents directly engaged in advocacy, policy making, and creating dialogue

Individual nurses at level 1 may be unaware of the need for nurses to unite or have accepted that nurses will not unite to support each other. Nurses at level 2 may be aware that a united nursing profession would be powerful but don't actively do anything to unite nurses. Level 1 nurses should first be made aware of the negative consequences of disunity within the nursing profession and actively take steps to unify them. All nursing schools should promote unification of the nursing profession as a core nursing value. Level 2 nurses should also actively seek to recognize what barriers (social, political, cultural, geographical, etc.) prevent them from helping nursing to be a more unified profession. These nurses should remove those barriers and actively take steps to unify the nursing profession by supporting and advocating for nurses and nursing issues beyond their specialty area.

Level	Individual Nurses
1, 2	Unite

Individual nurses at level 3 are minimally engaged in self-advocacy and at level 4 are moderately engaged. These nurses should learn the importance of unifying the nursing profession as well as take steps to become self-advocates beyond the bedside using a consistent and focused approach. These approaches may include consistent online and in-person activities to support nurses working in other specialty areas. Additionally, these nurses should challenge local professional organizations and labor unions to support other nurses who are not members of the organization or labor union.

Local nursing institutions, organizations, and labor unions may also be involved in promoting self-advocacy. Generally, and similar to individuals, these organizations should seek to understand the barriers preventing them from uniting with other local or national organizations. These organizations should seek to empower those nurses within their institution as well as the nurses in other organizations, specialty areas, and geographic locations. Finally, these organizations should use their platform to support not only the organizations that have similar philosophies and approaches to advocacy but also the organizations with different approaches. This support can be as simple as online activities to show solidarity or as complex as cooperating to hold in-person events, joining together politically behind a party, principle, or person. Regardless of how large or small these efforts are, they speak volumes to the nursing profession, all of healthcare, and the public. The message, "Nurses unequivocally support this initiative," is extremely powerful.

Specifically, I recommend the following for each kind of nursing organization. Professional nursing organizations have a reputation for advocating from ivory towers. These organizations could benefit from shifting that narrative to reflect one that is closer to the bedside and more in tune with the bedside nurse.

Local specialty nursing organizations could benefit from supporting each other and the general nursing profession by focusing some of their efforts on the issues that most nurses are concerned with. This empowers nurses and brings the power of specialty nursing organizations to the core battles nurses are having. Consolidating resources and power is essential. To quote Aristotle, the whole is greater than the sum of its parts.

In order to empower all nurses in the United States, nursing labor unions must move past the standard position of only supporting other labor unions. While this may be effective in some states, there are a considerable number of states where collective bargaining will not be an option for the foreseeable future. A nursing labor union only supporting other labor unions effectively disempowers the half of the population of nurses who cannot access this benefit in the United States. Nursing labor unions must actively support all nurses, regardless of their affiliation to the union or geographic location.

Level	Individual	Local Institutions
1, 2	Unite	Unite
3, 4		Empower

Level 5 nurses are highly engaged in self-advocacy, and level 6 nurses are high-level and powerful activists. Individuals at these levels are highly visible entrepreneurs, innovators, and leaders; create engagement opportunities for self and others; and seek out and engage issues. Similarly, organizations at this level are recognized nationally and some may be recognized internationally. Individuals and organizations at this level should lead the profession by unifying with each other to create nursing scientific consensus that addresses practice as well as local, national, and international problems. These individuals and organizations should be a beacon of light and hope. They have the influence and means to be an exemplar of how to support every nurse as well as each and every nursing organization. Importantly, these individuals and organizations can and should present as a unified front for the nursing profession and all who work in healthcare.

Finally, these individuals and organizations can help showcase the nursing profession in a big way when the world needs help. These individuals and organizations should use their collective resources and influence to "be the nursing response" to threats to health and well-being around the United States and the world. Additionally, a collective and unified response from all major players within the nursing profession means nurses are positioned to make a significant impact when a national or world event requires healthcare providers.

Level	Individual	Local Institutions	National and International Institutions
1, 2	Unite	Unite	Unite
3, 4		Empower	Empower
5, 6			Consensus

In conclusion, nurse self-advocacy beyond the bedside is the pathway to empowering nurses and transforming healthcare. The key conditions that nurses must work toward in order to manifest this destiny are unifying as individuals and professionals, empowering the entire nursing profession, and using nursing scientific consensus to guide advocacy efforts. The ladder of engagement can be used to determine where each individual nurse or nursing organization is in terms of their current self-advocacy efforts and offers a pathway to take those efforts to the next rung.

DISCUSSION AND REFLECTION POINTS

1. Regarding advocacy, what is your level of engagement?
2. What are the barriers (social, political, cultural, geographical, etc.) preventing you from helping unify nursing?
   a. What can you do about this?
3. Do you belong to a local nursing organization?
4. Do they support nurses outside the organization?
   a. If yes, how so?
   b. If no, why not?
5. What can you do to help nursing organizations support each other?
6. Name a national or international health crisis.
7. What national or international nursing organization is working on this?
8. What could be done differently to help this problem?

REFERENCES

Department for Professional Employees. (2019). *Safe staffing: Critical for patients and nurses* [Fact sheet 2019]. https://www.dpeaflcio.org/factsheets/safe-staffing-critical-for-patients-and-nurses

Massachusetts Nurses Association. (2001). *Massachusetts Nurses Association votes to disaffiliate from national organization, sets course for more progressive, pro-staff nurse agenda.* https://www.massnurses.org/news-and-events/archive/2001/p/openItem/2010

DISCUSSION AND REFLECTION POINTS

REFERENCES

The Future of Nursing and Healthcare

INTRODUCTION

I wrote this book because I was one of the frustrated nurses who left the bedside. I remember so many scary situations, too many close calls, and feeling like it was impossible to do my job the way I was trained to do it. I changed specialties. I changed settings. I earned advanced degrees. Nothing changed. The same issues followed me—being unsupported, feeling underappreciated for my work, high burnout, and dangerous clinical situations. Mostly, I felt I couldn't help people the way I was told I would be able to when I was in school. Despite all of that, choosing nursing for my profession saved my life in so many ways; it gave me purpose and helped me become a responsible contributing member of society. Despite the problems in our profession, I owe much of my good fortune to nursing. It is my hope and vision that each person who reads this book will take some small step toward improving nursing and that these collective steps will empower a nation of nurses to revolutionize all of healthcare.

This work, advocating for bedside nurses, has brought me back to the core of my profession and why I chose it to begin with. Bedside nurses are the largest workforce in healthcare. As nurses, we should not only be in control of our work environments; we must also have the autonomy to design them in a way so that we can care for our patients as we were trained to care for them. As nurses, we cannot allow money and greed to be the determining factor in how well we are able to care for our patients. If we believe that patients come before profits, we have to take a unified stand. We have to unify for our patients and for ourselves. I believe nurses should support nurses; nursing organizations should unify and consolidate their resources to address the core issues that nearly all nurses face; and, most important, we must unify to become the most powerful voices in the healthcare system.

I wrote this book for my patients, my family, my community, and my profession. I wrote this book because I may be a patient one day, and I want my nurse to have the best chance at caring for me, and maybe even saving my life. I wrote this book for you, because you may take care of patients now and you may also be a patient one day. We all deserve better.

This chapter is a summary of the previous six chapters as well as a discussion of a preferred future for nursing and healthcare. Additionally, this chapter is an invitation to readers to create a better future. This chapter is about a shared vision for nursing and healthcare and how using some simple methods, concepts, and principles can help nurses arrive at and operationalize this vision.

The preceding chapters describe nursing as an ailing entity, with symptoms and a cure. Regardless of whether or not this analogy resonates, the professional and systemic problems with nursing and healthcare are palpable and consequential. There are many methods and tools available to help nurses to lead and innovate within healthcare. Storytelling is a powerful method every nurse can use to capture the attention of other professionals as well as lay-people. The story of self, story of us, and story of now is a format every nurse can use to tell their story, or any nurs-ing-related story, and greatly improve the impact of their story. Every nurse can adopt this method of conveying their truth and, in doing so, can amplify the long-standing public trust in nurses into a purposeful public following and part-nership. In order to revolutionize healthcare, nurses require trust, as well as action, from the public. Corporations, as powerful as they are, cannot compete with the power of authentic human storytelling. In order for nurses to take more control within the healthcare industry, we must tell our stories boldly, loudly, and without reservation. Social media and the age of information allows every nurse to tell their story. Every nurse should know their story and tell it strategically.

Moving Forward

The ladder of engagement is a tool that can be used to propel the entire nursing profession forward. As a tool, the ladder of engagement is imperfect. However, concep-tually, every nurse and every nursing organization can use the ladder to propel themselves upward toward a more engaging, and more impactful, place within nurs-ing and healthcare. The concept is simple: Construct the ladder, determine where you are on the ladder, and move to the next rung of engagement. Determine the frequency of self-evaluation and repeat these steps. This book out-lines several steps, big and small, that every nurse can take to be a more impactful member of the nursing com-munity. I estimate that less than 3% of nurses are directly involved in self-advocacy beyond the bedside. The ladder of engagement allows every nurse, regardless of how engaged they are in self-advocacy, to become a little more engaged. If every nurse became slightly more involved in self-advocacy, nurses would revolutionize healthcare by sheer numbers alone. One way for nurses to revolutionize healthcare is for each nurse to find themselves on the ladder of engagement and then for every nurse to move up one rung.

Representation

An important culture change that can empower the nursing profession is to increase the representation and voice of nurses in the public view. Nurses can do this by using social media platforms to tell their stories publicly, refute unrealistic or stereotypical depictions of nurses, and ensure that there is accurate representation of nurses in media. Additionally, nurses should reflect to the public the nurse view of how to solve problems in the world. This nurse view should be based on scientific evidence and will ultimately reassure the public that nurses are more than trustworthy mothering types. This will demonstrate to the public that nurses are also a diverse group of professionals who adhere to and are guided by scientific principles. This standard also removes many reasons why nurses are not unified. A profession guided by science is a profession united by science.

Finally, we must increase the number of nurses at all political levels (institutional, state, federal, etc.). Nurses cannot assert influence without representation in the halls of power. Every nurse should use the ladder of engagement to assert themselves politically. Nurses running for public office should use scientific evidence as their rationale for their political positions. All nurses should support nurses seeking leadership opportunities or public office.

Similarly, every nursing organization should use their influence to endorse and support all political candidates who are nurses. Organizations should support these nurses regardless of political affiliation; if nurses are using science and evidence to drive policy, their political affiliation should not matter. An important cultural shift is necessary for nurses to become powerful within healthcare: Nurses must support nurses politically. Nurses who unify politically should use models and strategies like the snowflake model (Chapter 2) to form micro voting blocs. Nurses should also use their good standing and influence within their communities to form macro voting blocs, which can be used to drive nurse-centric policy and values to improve healthcare, government, and society at large.

Nursing Education

Nursing education has certainly come a long way. Still, there are structural and systemic problems that contribute to the dysfunction within the nursing profession. The hierarchy of healthcare and nursing is especially problematic. These education hierarchies fuel disunity and dysfunction and initiate students on a long path of political rivalry with fellow nurses.

First and foremost, the nurse educator shortage should be addressed by compensating nurses in academia based on their level of expertise and value added to the institution. Highly educated nurses should not take a pay cut to train the next generation of nurses. Second, all nursing higher education requires a complete overhaul and cultural change regarding hierarchical views of fellow nurses. The term "just a nurse" is ridiculous in that it downplays the education, experience, and intelligence of a nurse. However, every nurse is a nurse and not necessarily better or more important than any other nurse. There is a culture within nursing that overtly pushes the idea that more education makes a better nurse, for instance, the belief that a doctorally prepared nurse is somehow superior to an LPN. A more educated nurse has different skills and information but they are not automatically a better nurse. This idea of more academically qualified nurses being better is a significant reason why nurses in different specialties do not support each other.

In order for nurses to revolutionize healthcare, this culture must stop, and stopping this culture begins in nursing academia. In order for nurses to truly unify, we must flatten the hierarchy within the profession. The new nursing culture should be that every nurse is a nurse and every nurse supports every other nurse.

The Nurse Culture

This hierarchy is related to lateral violence. Lateral violence, or bullying, is the elephant in the room of the nursing profession. Every nurse knows the detrimental effects of lateral violence (as a recipient or contributor), yet few are willing to take a real stance against the practice. This is a real opportunity for nurses to reverse, or completely change, a destructive part of nursing culture. The snowflake model gives every nurse an opportunity to create small groups of nurses against lateral violence, who are proponents of the new culture of nurse unity. Every nurse should start this culture shift and pull others into this new way to be a professional nurse. This is a cultural movement that must happen within nursing in order for nurses to become truly powerful within the healthcare industry. Each individual nurse is responsible for the success or failure of this culture change. Every nurse can make this change immediately.

The U.S. healthcare system is not built for nurses. It is built for health insurance companies, pharmaceutical companies, healthcare institutions like hospitals, and medical providers like physicians and advance practice providers (APRNs, PAs [physician assistants], midwives, etc.). This is hugely problematic because the nurse is considered a budgetary line item and is often treated as such. Bedside nurses do not create direct revenue for a hospital or healthcare institution. This model can be and should be challenged.

The only way to challenge this model and include nurses in the healthcare system in a way that makes them less of a liability and more of an asset is to challenge the accrediting bodies and lawmakers who decide how healthcare works. This kind of effort requires a unified body of individual nurses as well as nursing organizations. Individual nurses and nursing organizations should challenge the reimbursement system by holding those who control healthcare-accrediting bodies, as well as lawmakers, accountable. This requires concerted, highly coordinated efforts from individual nurses and nursing organizations. To position themselves as powerful within healthcare, nurses should know who the accrediting bodies of their institution (or specialty) are and how to access the nurses and other board members.

A Leader and an Advocate

Every nurse is a leader and an advocate at the bedside. However, in order to become truly revolutionary, nurses must lead beyond the bedside. This starts with understanding our individual preferred leadership style. Nurses also navigate personal obstacles that make work beyond the bedside less appealing, such as associated professional risks and competing personal or professional interests. These are real barriers to leadership beyond the bedside. The ladder of engagement discussed in Chapter 5 offers an opportunity for self-evaluation as well as some incremental steps each nurse can take to become more of a leader beyond the bedside. Similarly, nursing organizations, while seemingly very busy, can be all but absent in the lives of bedside nurses and, even worse, the public. These organizations have a real opportunity to lead nurses by seeing the full view of the healthcare industry while simultaneously being with the nurses at the bedside. Nursing organizations must meet bedside nurses at the bedside, both during difficult times and during times of calm. Importantly, nursing organizations should unify the entire nursing profession by publicly working together toward shared goals rather than fighting publicly (or privately) and working against each other's interest. Finally, nursing organizations have an opportunity to really show up on the national and world stages during health-related crises. This should be a priority and will help gain public and professional trust.

Nurse Unity

Finally, there are three conditions that are essential for self-advocacy beyond the bedside, empowering a nation of nurses, and revolutionizing healthcare. These conditions are (a) unifying the nursing profession, (b) removing dysfunctional aspects of nursing culture as well as the powerless culture, and (c) committing overwhelmingly to use science and evidence to drive policy, politics, and change. This entire book is about empowering nurses to take a step toward these three conditions, in preparation for nurses to assume greater power and control of their own collective destinies. In doing so, nurses will completely revolutionize healthcare for the better. Every nurse should assess their place on the ladder of engagement as it pertains to self-advocacy beyond the bedside as well as any barriers that may prevent them from ascending to the next rung.

My vision for the nursing profession is fairly simple: a unified nursing profession, where every nurse attempts to ascend to the next rung on the self-advocacy ladder of engagement. This amount of activity and movement—nearly five million unified healthcare professionals—will awaken a sleeping giant, empower nurses everywhere, and send shock waves through the healthcare industry. Nurses will be recognized as essential as well as a formidable unified community within healthcare. The industry will balance with the most trusted professionals at the helm. The boot of the healthcare lobbyists and healthcare insurance companies will be lifted from the necks of nurses. Nurses will have control over their practice environments and will practice the way they were taught in school. Health outcomes will improve when nurses have more control of the healthcare system. Patients will be happier. Most important, every person born in the healthcare system will meet a nurse under the best conditions. Every person who receives healthcare throughout their life will receive care under the best conditions, and every person who dies within a healthcare facility will do so under the best conditions possible. This is my vision for my practice, my profession, for healthcare and for healthcare communities everywhere.

DISCUSSION AND REFLECTION POINTS

These are some key takeaways from this book and some actions every nurse can take moving forward.

1. Our professional stories are powerful. A key to unlocking our power is to tell our stories to family, coworkers, officials, and the public. This is how we move public trust to public action on our behalf.

2. Each of us must find our place on the ladder of engagement and move to the next rung. The key to actualizing our power is for each nurse, regardless of how small they believe their contribution is, to move up a rung on the ladder of engagement. This is how we mobilize an entire workforce.

3. Use social media to address underrepresentation and misrepresentation. A united nursing profession is a powerful force, and social media platforms allow nurses to use their collective voice to shift public narrative.

4. Support science and evidence to address all problems. This is a way to unify a culturally very diverse nursing profession behind policy, political, and social initiatives.

5. All nurses should support every other nurse professionally, in politics and in leadership. Nurses can be powerful at the bedside and as constituents. To maximize our effect, we must create a professional culture with strong fraternity and solid principles.

6. Every nurse must know who controls healthcare and how to reach out to these entities directly. If we want to change our circumstances, we must individually and collectively focus our efforts in the direction that will yield results.

7. We must challenge the system that categorizes nurses as budgetary line items and move toward a system that is nurse centric or includes nursing care as a significant piece of the reimbursement model.

8. Every nurse is a leader. Lead at your own pace in your own way. Be effective in the way you can. Lean into your leadership style, maximize your effect and efforts, at the bedside and beyond.

9. Mitigate risk of self-advocacy beyond the bedside by choosing activities within your comfort level. We should self-advocate consistently but when we can and in the way we can.

   Support professional nursing organizations that unify the profession. This should be the baseline expectation for all nursing professional organizations. Nurses should join, sponsor, promote, and be encouraged by organizations to unify the nursing profession and lead healthcare.

Index

Printed in the United States
by Baker & Taylor Publisher Services